MCQs for FRCOphth Part 1

T0177635

MCQs for FRCOphth Part 1

Sohaib R. Rufai **BMBS, BMedSc, MRes, FInstLM**

Recipient of the RCOphth Ulverscroft David Owen Prize
NIHR Doctoral Fellow and Specialist Registrar in Ophthalmology
University of Leicester Ulverscroft Eye Unit
Leicester, UK; and
Great Ormond Street Hospital for Children
London, UK

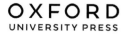

OXFORD
UNIVERSITY PRESS

OXFORD
UNIVERSITY PRESS

Great Clarendon Street, Oxford, OX2 6DP,
United Kingdom

Oxford University Press is a department of the University of Oxford.
It furthers the University's objective of excellence in research, scholarship,
and education by publishing worldwide. Oxford is a registered trade mark of
Oxford University Press in the UK and in certain other countries

© Oxford University Press 2023

The moral rights of the author have been asserted

First Edition published in 2023

Impression: 1

All rights reserved. No part of this publication may be reproduced, stored in
a retrieval system, or transmitted, in any form or by any means, without the
prior permission in writing of Oxford University Press, or as expressly permitted
by law, by licence or under terms agreed with the appropriate reprographics
rights organization. Enquiries concerning reproduction outside the scope of the
above should be sent to the Rights Department, Oxford University Press, at the
address above

You must not circulate this work in any other form
and you must impose this same condition on any acquirer

Published in the United States of America by Oxford University Press
198 Madison Avenue, New York, NY 10016, United States of America

British Library Cataloguing in Publication Data

Data available

Library of Congress Control Number: 2022946318

ISBN 978–0–19–284371–5

DOI: 10.1093/oso/9780192843715.001.0001

Printed and bound by
CPI Group (UK) Ltd, Croydon, CR0 4YY

Oxford University Press makes no representation, express or implied, that the
drug dosages in this book are correct. Readers must therefore always check
the product information and clinical procedures with the most up-to-date
published product information and data sheets provided by the manufacturers
and the most recent codes of conduct and safety regulations. The authors and
the publishers do not accept responsibility or legal liability for any errors in the
text or for the misuse or misapplication of material in this work. Except where
otherwise stated, drug dosages and recommendations are for the non-pregnant
adult who is not breast-feeding

Links to third party websites are provided by Oxford in good faith and
for information only. Oxford disclaims any responsibility for the materials
contained in any third party website referenced in this work.

DEDICATION

To my wonderful wife, Tania—this book was only possible due to your constant encouragement, love, and support. To my son, Adam—you are the light of my life. To my amazing parents—thank you for showing me the meaning of hard work and true love. To my sisters, brother-in-law, and wider family—thank you for always being there for me and encouraging me to work hard and dream big. To my colleagues, mentors, and patients, who teach me the art and science of ophthalmology. I humbly dedicate this book to you all.

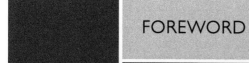

FOREWORD

Examinations are a necessary evil. I have yet to meet a student, young or old, who likes examinations. If one starts preparation too early, they cause chronic stress; if one leaves it until too late, they cause acute stress. Studying for examinations, even more than the actual examination, is part of the dislike. It detracts the student's time from the manifold other important things that occupy a student's life.

Yet, it is not easy to find anything else that gives a student more joy, more happiness, and a greater sense of achievement than passing an examination. This happiness is shared by their loved ones, making it even more special. And in the final reckoning, each successful examination stamps a mark of attainment that is indelible, sealing what has been attained and setting the student up for the next step along the career path. This makes examinations necessary and, dare I say, desirable.

So how does one balance this like–hate relationship? Different ways of studying work for different people. Early waking, late sleeping; individually or with friends; gradual and regular or short and intense studying (usually soon before an examination); seeking God's help through prayers and offerings; the list is endless. All working towards the same goal: accumulating, assimilating, and storing knowledge. The latter is called memory. Memory can be enhanced not so much by repeated reading but by proper understanding of the knowledge. 'That it is so' can be a piece of knowledge that one can learn by heart. Understanding 'Why is it so?' or 'How is it so?' makes it difficult to forget. Understanding brings another dimension to learning, the ability to synthesise knowledge and apply it to the question posed, be it by the patient's condition or by the examiner in a written or oral examination.

There is, however, another crucial aspect of successfully preparing for an examination—understanding the art of examination, which is not something one can pick up from the conventional sources of knowledge. Knowing what are the types of questions, the nuances contained within, the catchphrases where one can get caught out, what might appear to be asked versus what is being asked, and other such variations. This comes from practice and familiarity with the examination techniques and texts. This is where this resource, *MCQs for FRCOphth Part 1* by Dr Sohaib Rufai, becomes invaluable. It deals with the full range of topics covered in the Fellowship of the Royal College of Ophthalmologists (FRCOphth) Part 1 examination in the form of multiple-choice questions, which one can use to test one's knowledge. It familiarises the student with the phraseology used in the formulation of questions, indicates the correct answers, and provides the explanation for why they are right and the reasoning for why the incorrect answers are wrong. Just knowing the right answers would be useful if it were guaranteed that these were the questions that one would encounter in the examination. If only! The approach adopted in this book makes 'getting it wrong' a useful learning exercise. The author's youth makes the questions relevant and timely, the depth and breadth in age and experience of the dozen reviewers make the content valid and verified.

Reading this book will impart ready-packaged knowledge that can be applied to answer a range of questions. When the examination is imminent, this book will become a valuable tool for revision. Use it to revise and become wise.

Professor Harminder S. Dua, CBE

MBBS, DO, DO(London), MS, MNAMS, FRCS (Edinburgh), FEBO (EU), FRCOphth, FRCP (Edinburgh, Honorary), FCOptom (UK, Honorary), FRCOphth (UK, Honorary), MD, PhD

Former President of the Royal College of Ophthalmologists 2011–2014

Chair and Professor of Ophthalmology

University of Nottingham

Queens Medical Centre

Nottingham, UK

PREFACE

Through this book project, I have made it my personal mission to help you pass your FRCOphth Part 1 exam.

Preparing this book has highlighted the sheer vastness of the Part 1 syllabus. It is not possible to cover every single possible question and minute detail that could come up. Instead, it is best to aim for breadth and high-yield material to maximise your chances of exceeding the pass mark.

The full FRCOphth Part 1 exam details, syllabus, and previous exam reports are available via the Royal College of Ophthalmologists (RCOphth) website (www.rcophth.ac.uk)—I would encourage you to read these carefully.

The Part 1 exam covers the following core subjects: Optics, Anatomy, Physiology, Pathology, Pharmacology, Genetics, Investigations, and Miscellaneous (including biostatistics and evidence-based medicine), each with various categories and subcategories. Please note that the subject weighting and exam format have changed significantly in 2021, hence this book has been produced to reflect these new changes.

This book contains 450 multiple-choice questions (MCQs) with solutions, explanations, and recommended reading, weighted across the core subjects to reflect the typical breakdown from recent Part 1 exam reports. The 450 MCQs in this book are evenly spread across five chapters, or 'practice papers'. You can either work through them at your own pace to develop your knowledge, or use them as mock papers under exam conditions, or a combination of both. The actual exam consists of two MCQ papers featuring 90 questions each, with 2 hours to complete each paper.

I would recommend setting aside several months to systematically prepare for the exam and balance revision with your clinical work and home life. Reading material and practice questions should be used together and not in isolation. The RCOphth provides a recommended reading list online with core textbooks—some of the general textbooks require careful reading while other more specialised textbooks can simply be dipped into when the need arises. Consider preparing a timetable to set aside dedicated revision time per subject. Consider working with a partner or small group, in person or virtually, as this can keep you motivated, accountable to one another, and can promote effective peer teaching and learning. Identify how you learn best and use these methods to tackle new concepts, whether this is with short notes, lists, acronyms, mnemonics, drawings, ray diagrams, spider-diagrams, flashcards, or by other means—whatever works best for you.

This book may highlight knowledge gaps requiring broader and/or deeper reading and understanding. One can often diagnose the underlying problem by looking for patterns in the incorrect answers. If all questions across a category are answered incorrectly, the candidate needs to increase their breadth of knowledge. If questions within specific subcategories are answered incorrectly, the candidate may need to increase their depth of knowledge. If questions are answered inconsistently within the same category/subcategory, the candidate may need to work on exam technique. I hope this book serves as a useful tool to help tackle all of the above.

I am immensely grateful to all the reviewers for supporting this book project and carefully reviewing the MCQs and solutions in their areas of expertise. I am particularly grateful to Professor Harminder Dua for endorsing this book and writing the foreword. I also wish to thank all my colleagues who contributed high-quality figures to further aid learning.

I wish you all the very best for your exams, successful careers, good health, and happiness.

Sohaib R. Rufai

ACKNOWLEDGEMENTS

Reviewers

Mr Richard Bowman Consultant Paediatric Ophthalmologist, Great Ormond Street Hospital for Children, London, UK

Dr Catey Bunce Consultant in Applied Medical Statistics, Royal Marsden, London, UK

Professor Harold Ellis Professor of Anatomy and Emeritus Professor of Surgery, King's College London, UK

Ms Sri Gore Consultant Paediatric Ophthalmologist, Great Ormond Street Hospital for Children, London, UK

Professor Irene Gottlob Emeritus Professor of Ophthalmology, University of Leicester Ulverscroft Eye Unit, UK

Professor I. Christopher Lloyd Consultant Paediatric Ophthalmologist, Great Ormond Street Hospital for Children, London, UK

Professor Omar Mahroo Professor of Retinal Neuroscience, UCL Institute of Ophthalmology and Moorfields Eye Hospital, London, UK

Dr Hardeep Singh Mudhar Consultant Ophthalmic Pathologist, National Specialist Ophthalmic Pathology Service, Royal Hallamshire Hospital, Sheffield, UK

Ms Ameenat Lola Solebo NIHR Clinician Scientist and Honorary Consultant Paediatric Ophthalmologist, UCL Great Ormond Street Institute of Child Health, London, UK

Ms Lynne Speedwell Head of Optometry, Great Ormond Street Hospital for Children, London, UK

Mr Mervyn G. Thomas NIHR Academic Clinical Lecturer in Ophthalmology and Genomic Medicine, University of Leicester Ulverscroft Eye Unit, UK

Dr Dorothy A. Thompson Consultant Clinical Scientist, Great Ormond Street Hospital for Children, London, UK

Special thanks

I would like to thank the following colleagues for providing figures. Dr Tania Aslam Rufai, GP Registrar, Kent, for agreeing to be the 'eye model' for the book cover and various images within this book. Mr Syed Riyaz Ahmad, retired ophthalmologist, Essex, for providing anatomy illustrations. Mr Umar Ahmed, Medical Student at Imperial College London, for providing optics ray diagrams and numerous other schematics. Mr Aswin Chari, Clinical Research Fellow in Neurosurgery, Great Ormond Street Hospital for Children (GOSH), for providing neuroimaging figures. Dr Hardeep Singh Mudhar, Consultant Ophthalmic Pathologist at Royal Hallamshire Hospital, for providing histopathological images. Mr Dermot F. Roche, Vision Scientist at GOSH, for performing specialist ophthalmic imaging. Dr Dorothy Thompson, Consultant Clinical Scientist at GOSH, for providing electrodiagnostic diagrams. Finally, thank you to Oxford University Press for publishing this book.

CONTENTS

ABBREVIATIONS

AI   artificial intelligence
AMD   age-related macular degeneration
AV   atrioventricular
BCC   basal cell carcinoma
D   dioptre
ECG   electrocardiogram
EOG   electro-oculogram
ERG   electroretinogram
exo   exoenzyme
FFA   fundus fluorescein angiography
ffERG   full-field electroretinogram
FRCOphth   Fellowship of the Royal College of Ophthalmologists
GAG   glycosaminoglycan
H&E   haematoxylin and eosin
HLA   human leukocyte antigen
ICD-11   International Classification of Diseases, 11th revision
ICG   indocyanine green
IOL   intraocular lens
IOP   intraocular pressure
LP:DT   light peak:dark trough
MCQ   multiple-choice question
mgERG   multifocal electroretinogram
MRI   magnetic resonance imaging
Nd-YAG   neodymium–yttrium aluminium garnet
OCT   optical coherence tomography
OCTA   optical coherence tomography angiography
PAL   progressive addition lens
PCR   polymerase chain reaction
PERG   pattern electroretinogram
POAG   primary open-angle glaucoma
prVEP   pattern reversal visual evoked potential

RAPD	relative afferent pupillary defect
RPE	retinal pigment epithelium
RSM	relative spectacle magnification
SIGN	Scottish Intercollegiate Guidelines Network
SLO	scanning laser ophthalmoscopy
UBM	ultrasound biomicroscopy
US	ultrasonography
VEP	visual evoked potential

QUESTIONS

Optics 1

1. **Which of the following ranges represent the visible wavelengths of the electromagnetic spectrum, in nanometres (nm)?**
    A. 400–780 nm
    B. 500–880 nm
    C. 600–980 nm
    D. 700–1080 nm

2. **Regarding the intensity of light, which statement is MOST likely to be correct?**
    A. Radiant intensity is measured in joules and luminous intensity is measured in lumens.
    B. Radiant intensity is measured in lumens and luminous energy is measured in joules.
    C. Radiant intensity is measured in watts per steradian and luminous intensity is measured in candelas.
    D. Radiant intensity is measured in candelas and luminous intensity is measured in watts per steradian.

3. **Which of the following represents the image formed by a concave mirror where the object lies outside the centre of curvature?**
    A. Image real, inverted, enlarged
    B. Image virtual, erect, enlarged
    C. Image real, inverted, diminished
    D. Image real, erect, enlarged

4. **Which of the following utilises total internal reflection?**
    A. Fibreoptic cable
    B. Volk 90-dioptre lens
    C. Fresnel prism
    D. Focimeter

MCQs for FRCOphth Part 1. Sohaib R. Rufai, Oxford University Press. © Oxford University Press 2023.
DOI: 10.1093/oso/9780192843715.003.0001

5. **What is the lens power of a ×8 loupe?**
   A. 4 dioptres
   B. 8 dioptres
   C. 16 dioptres
   D. 32 dioptres

6. **Which of the following represents the correct transposition of this lens prescription?**

   $$\frac{+3.00\ DS}{+1.50\ DC}\ axis\ 100$$

   A. $\dfrac{+3.25\ DS}{-1.50\ DC}\ axis\ 100$

   B. $\dfrac{+4.50\ DS}{+1.50\ DC}\ axis\ 10$

   C. $\dfrac{+4.50\ DS}{-1.50\ DC}\ axis\ 10$

   D. $\dfrac{+3.25\ DS}{-1.50\ DC}\ axis\ 100$

7. **In Gullstrand's schematic eye, what is the distance of the second nodal point behind the anterior corneal surface, in millimetres?**
   A. 7.08
   B. 7.18
   C. 7.33
   D. 7.43

8. **Regarding hypermetropia, which statement is LEAST likely to be correct?**
   A. Manifest hypermetropia is defined as the strongest concave lens correction accepted for clear distance vision.
   B. Latent hypermetropia is masked by ciliary tone and involuntary accommodation.
   C. Hypermetropia that can be overcome by accommodation is termed facultative.
   D. Hypermetropia exceeding the amplitude of accommodation is termed absolute.

9. **Which of the following does NOT represent an optical problem when correcting aphakia with spectacles?**
   A. Ring scotomas
   B. Jack-in-the-box phenomenon
   C. Heavy lenses
   D. Barrel distortion

10. **Regarding bifocal lenses, which statement is LEAST likely to be true?**

A. Excessive prismatic effect at the near visual point can be particularly marked in high-powered lenses.

B. Prismatic jump can be minimised if the optical centres of the two lenses lie away from the junction of the distance and near portions.

C. Split bifocals represent the earliest bifocal design.

D. Solid bifocals are those of single-piece construction.

11. **Which of the following does NOT represent a stage within retinoscopy?**

A. Illumination stage

B. Dark-adaptation stage

C. Reflex stage

D. Projection stage

12. **Regarding the Javal–Schiøtz keratometer, which statement is MOST likely to be true?**

A. The instrument uses an object of fixed size.

B. Each mire is a small lantern with a clear window.

C. Doubling of the image is achieved using a Porro prism.

D. When examining an astigmatic patient, the two images are displaced vertically in all except the two principal meridians of the cornea.

13. **Regarding lenses for fundus examination, which statement is MOST likely to be true?**

A. The Hruby lens is a powerful plano-convex lens.

B. The 90-dioptre lens provides more magnification than the 78-dioptre lens.

C. The panfunduscope contact lens forms a virtual, inverted image of the fundus.

D. The field of view of the 78-dioptre lens is less than that achieved by the panfunduscope contact lens.

14. **What does the acronym 'LASER' stand for?**

A. Laser Amplification by Stimulated Energy Radiation

B. Light Amplification by Stimulated Energy Radiation

C. Laser Amplification by Stimulated Emission of Radiation

D. Light Amplification by Stimulated Emission of Radiation

15. **Regarding auto-refractors, which statement is LEAST likely to be true?**

A. All but infrared light is filtered out.

B. The fixation target is designed to avoid accommodation by the patient.

C. The instrument detects the end point of refraction using an electronic focus detector.

D. The instrument performs well even in eyes with broad iridectomies.

16. **Regarding slit lamp filters, which statement is LEAST likely to be correct?**
    A. Red light is scattered more than blue light.
    B. The cobalt blue filter is used for applanation tonometry.
    C. The green (red-free) filter is useful for inspecting the vitreous.
    D. Blue light is of 465–490 nanometres.

Anatomy 1

17. **Regarding walls of the orbit, which statement is MOST likely to be true?**
    A. The roof comprises the orbital plate of frontal bone and body of sphenoid.
    B. The floor comprises the orbital plate of maxilla, orbital surface of zygomatic, and orbital process of palatine.
    C. The lateral wall comprises the zygomatic bone and lesser wing of sphenoid.
    D. The medial wall comprises the frontal process of maxilla, lacrimal bone, orbital plate of ethmoid, and greater wing of sphenoid.

18. **Regarding the eyelids, which statement is LEAST likely to be true?**
    A. The insertion of the aponeurotic fibres of the levator palpebrae superioris forms the upper eyelid sulcus.
    B. The malar and nasojugal sulci may be present in older individuals.
    C. When the eye is closed, the upper eyelid normally covers the upper half of the cornea.
    D. The superior palpebral sulcus divides each eyelid into an orbital and tarsal part.

19. **Regarding the orbicularis oculi muscle, which statement is LEAST likely to be true?**
    A. The orbicularis oculi muscle is supplied by temporal and zygomatic branches of the seventh cranial nerve.
    B. The action of the palpebral portion is both voluntary and involuntary.
    C. The fibres of the palpebral portion sweep concentrically and laterally across the lids, behind the orbital septum.
    D. The lacrimal portion draws the eyelids and papillae medially.

20. **Which nerve does NOT pass through the common tendinous ring?**
    A. Nasociliary
    B. Abducent
    C. Trochlear
    D. Upper division of oculomotor

21. **Where does the optic nerve perforate the sclera, in millimetres (mm)?**
    A. 3 mm medial and 1 mm above the posterior pole
    B. 1 mm medial and 3 mm above the posterior pole
    C. 3 mm lateral and 1 mm below the posterior pole
    D. 1 mm lateral and 3 mm below the posterior pole

22. **Regarding the cornea, which statement is LEAST likely to be true?**
    A. The central cornea is supplied with oxygen dissolved in the tear film.
    B. The peripheral cornea is supplied with oxygen by diffusion from the posterior ciliary blood vessels.
    C. The long ciliary nerves provide sensory innervation to the cornea.
    D. Complete turnover of the surface epithelial cells is estimated to take 7 days.

23. **Regarding the pituitary fossa, which statement is MOST likely to be true?**
    A. It is formed by an indentation in the ethmoid bone.
    B. It is anteriorly bound by the dorsum sellae.
    C. It is posteriorly bound by the tuberculum sellae.
    D. It is roofed by the diaphragma sella.

24. **Which of the following options represents the correct order of layers of the retina, from inner to outer layers?**
    A. Internal limiting membrane, nerve fibre layer, ganglion cell layer, inner plexiform layer, outer plexiform layer, inner nuclear layer, outer nuclear layer, external limiting membrane, ellipsoid zone, retinal pigment epithelium
    B. Internal limiting membrane, nerve fibre layer, ganglion cell layer, inner nuclear layer, outer nuclear layer, inner plexiform layer, outer plexiform layer, external limiting membrane, ellipsoid zone, retinal pigment epithelium
    C. Internal limiting membrane, nerve fibre layer, ganglion cell layer, inner plexiform layer, inner nuclear layer, outer plexiform layer, outer nuclear layer, external limiting membrane, ellipsoid zone, retinal pigment epithelium
    D. Internal limiting membrane, nerve fibre layer, ganglion cell layer, inner plexiform layer, outer plexiform layer, inner nuclear layer, outer nuclear layer, ellipsoid zone, retinal pigment epithelium, external limiting membrane

25. **Approximately how long is the intracranial portion of the optic nerve, in millimetres (mm)?**
    A. 1 mm
    B. 5 mm
    C. 10 mm
    D. 25 mm

26. **Which of the following represents the correct order of structures of the anterior chamber angle as seen on gonioscopy, from posterior to anterior?**

A. Iris, ciliary body, scleral spur, Schwalbe's line, trabecular meshwork
B. Iris, scleral spur, ciliary body, Schwalbe's line, trabecular meshwork
C. Iris, ciliary body, scleral spur, trabecular meshwork, Schwalbe's line
D. Iris, scleral spur, ciliary body, trabecular meshwork, Schwalbe's line

27. **Regarding classification of the extraocular muscles, which statement is LEAST likely to be true?**

A. Type B muscle fibres possess a smaller diameter than type A muscle fibres.
B. Type C muscle fibres align both visual axes with fine local contractions.
C. Type B muscle fibres possess multiple end plates.
D. Type A muscle fibres are mainly involved in smooth pursuit movements.

28. **What is the secondary action of the superior oblique muscle?**

A. Intorsion
B. Extorsion
C. Abduction
D. Adduction

29. **Regarding the lateral geniculate nucleus, which statement is LEAST likely to be true?**

A. It is located on the undersurface of the pulvinar of the thalamus.
B. It receives the caudal termination of the lateral root of the optic tract.
C. The contralateral eye sends visual information to layers 2, 3, and 5 of the lateral geniculate nucleus.
D. Its inner two layers are magnocellular layers, while its outer four layers are parvocellular layers.

30. **On what day of embryological development can the lens placode be identified?**

A. 27
B. 30
C. 37
D. 40

Physiology 1

Physiology of the eye and vision

31. What is the approximate thickness of the precorneal tear film in micrometres (μm)?

A. 3.4 μm
B. 6.8 μm
C. 13.4 μm
D. 16.8 μm

32. Which of the following represents the unconventional outflow pathway of aqueous humour at the anterior chamber angle?

A. Trabecular meshwork, collector channels, Schlemm's canal, aqueous veins, episcleral venous circulation
B. Trabecular meshwork, Schlemm's canal, collector channels, aqueous veins, episcleral venous circulation
C. Iris root, uveal meshwork, ciliary muscle, suprachoroidal space, sclera
D. Iris root, ciliary muscle, uveal meshwork, suprachoroidal space, sclera

33. What shaped suture is formed by the lens fibres meeting posteriorly?

A. Y
B. V
C. Inverted Y
D. Inverted V

34. What is the resting membrane potential of a dark-adapted rod cell, in millivolts (mV)?

A. −40 mV
B. −70 mV
C. −100 mV
D. −130 mV

35. Regarding visual acuity, which statement is LEAST likely to be true?

A. Visual acuity testing measures an individual's ability to discriminate two stimuli separated in space.
B. Bloch's law assumes a monotonic decrease in perceived contrast with increased duration.
C. The Broca–Sulzer effect assumes a peak in perceived contrast with prolonged duration.
D. At 5° from the central fovea, visual acuity drops to 25% of foveal acuity.

36. **Regarding the pupillary light reflex, which statement is MOST likely to be true?**
    A. The pupillary light reflex varies the amount of retinal illumination in response to changes in lighting.
    B. Pupil input from retinal ganglion cells leaves the optic tract in the brachium of the inferior colliculus.
    C. Neurons in the olivary pretectal nucleus send crossed and uncrossed fibres via the posterior commissure to the Edinger–Westphal nucleus.
    D. Postganglionic parasympathetic neurons pass from the ciliary ganglion via the long ciliary nerves to the iris sphincter muscle.

37. **Deutan defects are most commonly associated with the absence of which gene?**
    A. *OPN1DW*
    B. *OPN1SW*
    C. *OPN1LW*
    D. *OPN1MW*

General physiology

38. **Regarding action potentials, which statement is MOST likely to be true?**
    A. There is a positive membrane potential present during the resting stage.
    B. During depolarisation, the nerve fibre membrane becomes permeable to sodium ions.
    C. The potassium channels close during the repolarisation stage.
    D. In smaller nerve fibres and many central nervous system neurons, the membrane potential overshoots above the zero level during depolarisation.

39. **Regarding cardiac arrhythmias, which statement is MOST likely to be true?**
    A. Tachycardia is defined as a heart rate faster than 90 beats per minute.
    B. Second-degree type II atrioventricular (AV) block is characterised by a progressive prolongation of the PR interval until a ventricular beat is skipped.
    C. Third-degree AV block typically features a fixed number of non-conducted P waves per QRS complex.
    D. Atrial fibrillation reduces the efficiency of ventricular pumping by 20–30%.

40. **Regarding sensory receptors, which of the following does NOT cause receptor potentials?**
    A. Application of a chemical
    B. Effects of electromagnetic radiation
    C. Closure of ion channels
    D. Mechanical deformation

41. Which of the following hormones is NOT secreted by the anterior pituitary gland?

A. Prolactin

B. Oxytocin

C. Thyroid-stimulating hormone

D. Growth hormone

Biochemistry

42. Regarding the nucleus, which statement is LEAST likely to be true?

A. The nuclear membrane contains receptors for ligands.

B. Heterochromatin is less packed than euchromatin.

C. Chromatin is the main nuclear component.

D. The nucleolus is the site of ribosomal RNA synthesis and substantial transcriptional activity.

43. Regarding the biochemical properties of the vitreous, which statement is LEAST likely to be true?

A. Collagen type II is predominantly responsible for the gel structure of the vitreous body.

B. The central vitreous body possesses a higher concentration of hyaluronan and collagen as compared to the cortex.

C. Floaters become visible with age when the hyaluronan molecules degrade into smaller moieties while the collagen fibrils coagment, forming larger fibrils.

D. Opticin possesses a role in regulating fibril thickness within the vitreous body.

Pathology 1

General and ocular pathology

44. Regarding acute inflammation, which statement is MOST likely to be correct?

A. Following transendothelial migration and extravasation, the movement of leucocytes is subsequently controlled by expression.

B. Chemotactic agents are released from cytokines, complement components, leukotrienes, or pathogenic bacteria.

C. Phagocytosis involves opsonisation of bacteria by leucocytes followed by engulfment within complement components.

D. Histamine and leukotrienes decrease vascular permeability.

45. Regarding the healing and repair of ocular structures, which statement is LEAST likely to be correct?

A. Following trauma, reactive proliferation of the iris pigment epithelium may take place.

B. Scar tissue in the sclera is derived from scleral fibroblasts.

C. Axonal loss and demyelination occur following trauma to the optic nerve.

D. The limbus is the site at which the corneal epithelium regenerates.

46. Regarding cataractogenesis, which statement is LEAST likely to be true?

A. Lens crystallins break down to albuminoids.

B. Amino acids are converted to adrenaline and melanin.

C. There is reduced absorption of blue light.

D. Nuclear sclerosis and loss of zonule elasticity contribute to presbyopia.

47. Regarding Sjögren's syndrome, which statement is LEAST likely to be true?

A. Individuals with primary Sjögren's syndrome possess specific antibodies (anti-Rho, anti-La).

B. Xerostomia is a prevalent clinical feature.

C. Affected glands include the glands of Wolfring and Krause.

D. There is a proliferation of goblet cells in the conjunctival epithelium.

48. Regarding vitelliform dystrophy, which statement is LEAST likely to be true?

A. Classic fundoscopic findings include an egg-yolk lesion with satellite lesions.

B. Peripherin 2 is required for normal photoreceptor function.

C. Vitelliform macular dystrophy is caused by mutations in *BEST1* and *PRPH2*.

D. There is an accumulation of lipofuscin in the outer nuclear layer and atrophy of the photoreceptor layer.

49. Which of the following stains is most useful for identifying macular corneal dystrophy?

A. Oil Red O

B. Masson trichrome

C. Alcian blue

D. Congo red

50. Regarding herpes simplex keratitis, which statement is MOST likely to be true?

A. Type 1 herpes simplex virus can cause dendritic ulceration within the corneal endothelium.

B. Primary infection rarely occurs through the oral mucosa.

C. Complications of herpes simplex infection of the eye include disciform keratitis and secondary lipid keratopathy.

D. When reactivated, the virus can produce vesicle formation in the skin.

51. Which of the following does NOT represent a common primary site for choroidal metastasis?

A. Lung

B. Brain

C. Prostate

D. Breast

Microbiology

52. **Approximately what proportion of total white cells is constituted by neutrophils, in normal individuals?**
    A. 15%
    B. 25%
    C. 35%
    D. 45%

53. **What is the MOST common cause of postoperative pseudophakic endophthalmitis?**
    A. *Staphylococcus epidermidis*
    B. *Escherichia coli*
    C. *Propionibacterium acnes*
    D. *Staphylococcus aureus*

54. **What type of parasite is *Toxocara canis*?**
    A. Trematode
    B. Nematode
    C. Cestode
    D. Protozoan

Immunology

55. **Which of the following is NOT a cell of the mononuclear phagocyte system?**
    A. Eosinophils
    B. Dendritic cells
    C. Macrophages
    D. Monocytes

56. **Regarding human leukocyte antigen (HLA) associations, which statement is MOST likely to be true?**
    A. HLA-B51 is associated with ankylosing spondylitis.
    B. HLA-DR4 is associated with Vogt–Koyanagi–Harada disease.
    C. HLA-B27 is associated with birdshot retinochoroidopathy.
    D. HLA-A29 is associated with Behçet's retinal vasculitis.

Pharmacology and genetics 1

Pharmacology

57. Which law can predict the rate of diffusion though a cell membrane?

  A. Fick's law
  B. Sherrington's law
  C. Frank–Starling law
  D. Poiseuille's law

58. What is the approximate natural tear volume, in microlitres (µL)?

  A. 1–2 µL
  B. 7–8 µL
  C. 15–16 µL
  D. 24–25 µL

59. Which of the following sympathomimetics is an α_2 partial agonist?

  A. Phenylephrine
  B. Apraclonidine
  C. Brimonidine
  D. Cocaine

60. Regarding the properties of local anaesthetics, which statement is MOST likely to be true?

  A. They are inactivated in the plasma and liver by non-specific esterases.
  B. The pH of local anaesthetic is unaltered by the addition of adrenaline solution.
  C. They comprise an amide residue linked to a basic side chain.
  D. The amide group is hydrophobic.

61. Which of the following biologic agents is NOT a humanised monoclonal antibody?

  A. Adalimumab
  B. Infliximab
  C. Rituximab
  D. Tocilizumab

62. Regarding adrenergic agonists, which statement is LEAST likely to be true?

  A. Brimonidine is a non-selective α-receptor antagonist.
  B. Apraclonidine hydrochloride is a selective α_2-receptor agonist.
  C. Timolol is a non-selective β-blocker.
  D. Phenylephrine acts directly on α-receptors.

Genetics

63. **Which of the following represents the correct order of the stages of mitosis?**
   A. Prophase, metaphase, telophase, anaphase
   B. Prophase, anaphase, metaphase, telophase
   C. Prophase, anaphase, telophase, metaphase
   D. Prophase, metaphase, anaphase, telophase

64. **Which syndrome is associated with trisomy 18?**
   A. Patau
   B. Klinefelter
   C. Down
   D. Edwards

65. **Regarding mitochondrial inheritance, which statement is LEAST likely to be true?**
   A. Inheritance is exclusively maternal.
   B. Males and females can receive the defective gene.
   C. The acrosome of the sperm is conserved during fertilisation.
   D. Mitochondrial DNA replicates independently of the nuclear genome.

66. **Which of the following gene mutations is associated with Axenfeld–Rieger syndrome?**
   A. *FOXC1*
   B. *PAX6*
   C. *RS1*
   D. *RB1*

67. **Regarding gene therapy principles, which statement is LEAST likely to be true?**
   A. The gene gun is an efficient way to inject naked DNA.
   B. The coding DNA is often flanked by regulatory sequences.
   C. Vectors can be used to facilitate cell entry of DNA.
   D. Optogenetic therapy does not require replacement of the gene in question.

68. **Regarding candidate gene analysis, which statement is LEAST likely to be true?**
   A. Candidate genes expressed by the tissue in question are identified.
   B. A gene marker in the human genome close to the culprit gene defect is identified.
   C. Patients are screened for mutations in candidate genes.
   D. Candidate gene analysis does not require knowledge of the functions of proteins from the genes in question.

Investigations 1

69. **When performing the Maddox rod test on a patient with right exophoria, if the Maddox rod is positioned horizontally in front of the right eye fixing on a white spot of light, where will the red line appear?**
    A. Straight through the white spot
    B. To the left of the white spot
    C. To the right of the white spot
    D. Above the white spot

70. **Regarding the cover test, upon covering the right eye, what is indicated by inward turning of the uncovered left eye to fix on a target?**
    A. Left exotropia
    B. Left esotropia
    C. Left exophoria
    D. Left esophoria

71. **Which of the following visual field defects is MOST likely to be caused by papilloedema?**
    A. Pie in the sky
    B. Pie on the floor
    C. Central scotoma
    D. Blind spot enlargement

72. **Regarding keratometry, which statement is MOST likely to be true?**
    A. Curvature of the entire corneal surface is mapped.
    B. It is expressed as two corneal curvature values, 45° apart.
    C. It can be performed by the IOLMaster® device.
    D. It cannot be performed by autorefractors.

73. **Which of the following is LEAST likely to represent a relative contraindication to fundus fluorescein angiography?**
    A. Fluorescein allergy
    B. Shellfish allergy
    C. Renal impairment
    D. Pregnancy

74. **Regarding indocyanine green (ICG) angiography, which statement is MOST likely to be true?**
   A. ICG is 50% bound to serum proteins that do not pass through choriocapillaris vessel fenestrations.
   B. ICG emits light at 830 nm.
   C. Window defect is commonly caused by choroidal haemangioma.
   D. ICG angiography is safe in pregnancy.

75. **Regarding optical coherence tomography angiography (OCTA), which statement is MOST likely to be true?**
   A. It requires an intravenous contrast agent.
   B. It delivers lower resolution than fundus fluorescein angiography.
   C. It is more prone to artefact than fundus fluorescein angiography.
   D. It is more time-consuming to perform than fundus fluorescein angiography.

76. **Approximately what is the axial resolution of ocular ultrasound, in micrometres (μm)?**
   A. 5 μm
   B. 50 μm
   C. 100 μm
   D. 150 μm

77. **Regarding pachymetry, which statement is LEAST likely to be true?**
   A. A 20 MHz ultrasonic probe is used.
   B. Average central corneal thickness is between 490 and 560 micrometres.
   C. Intraocular pressure is underestimated in patients with thick corneas.
   D. Pachymetry can assess risk of postoperative ectasia prior to laser refractive surgery.

78. **Regarding the pattern reversal visual evoked potential (VEP), in a normal subject, when would the positive deflection be expected?**
   A. 50 milliseconds
   B. 75 milliseconds
   C. 100 milliseconds
   D. 135 milliseconds

79. **Regarding the visual evoked potential (VEP), which statement is MOST likely to be true?**
   A. Pattern reversal VEP is useful in patients with limited cooperation.
   B. In pattern reversal VEP, positive deflection occurs at 50 milliseconds.
   C. Trans-occipital crossed asymmetry can occur in albinism.
   D. There is one negative deflection.

Miscellaneous 1

80. **Regarding hypothesis testing, which statement is MOST likely to be true?**
    A. The p-value represents the probability that the null hypothesis is false.
    B. A type II error occurs where the null hypothesis is incorrectly accepted.
    C. Power is equal to 1 minus the probability of a type I error.
    D. A power of 70% is generally considered acceptable in study design.

81. **Which reporting guideline should be used for systematic reviews?**
    A. CONSORT
    B. STROBE
    C. STARD
    D. PRISMA

82. **Likert scales produce which type of data?**
    A. Nominal
    B. Ordinal
    C. Binary
    D. Continuous

83. **What is the modal value of the following numbers?**
    54, 60, 48, 34, 34, 40, 48, 31, 54, 52, 48
    A. 54
    B. 48
    C. 34
    D. 40

84. **In a study comparing one glaucoma treatment in one group of patients to another glaucoma treatment in a separate group of patients, where the outcome is intraocular pressure and the data are normally distributed, what is the MOST appropriate statistical test to use?**
    A. Paired t-test
    B. Unpaired t-test
    C. Wilcoxon signed rank test
    D. Mann–Whitney U test

85. **What is the MOST appropriate statistical test to use when the outcome measure is categorical and the data are paired?**
    A. Mann–Whitney U test
    B. Wilcoxon signed rank test
    C. Chi-squared test
    D. McNemar's test

86. **What is the MOST appropriate statistical test to use for three groups where the outcome measure is continuous and the data are skewed?**
    A. Analysis of variation
    B. Wilcoxon signed rank test
    C. Kruskal–Wallis test
    D. Fisher's exact test

87. **Which of the following options is MOST likely to lead to recall bias?**
    A. The tendency to search for or favour information that confirms prior beliefs
    B. Differences in the accuracy or completeness of recollections by participants regarding past events
    C. Unequal loss of participants from different arms of a trial
    D. Failure to achieve proper randomisation during participant selection

88. **A team of researchers have developed an artificial intelligence (AI)-assisted software to diagnose dry age-related macular degeneration (AMD) in the community. Their study results are displayed in the following 2 × 2 table:**

	AMD present	AMD absent
AI software positive	90	20
AI software negative	10	180

I. What is the positive predictive value of the AI-assisted software in detecting AMD, in per cent and to the nearest whole number?
   A. 80%
   B. 82%
   C. 90%
   D. 95%

II. What is the negative predictive value of the AI-assisted software in detecting AMD, in per cent and to the nearest whole number?
   A. 80%
   B. 82%
   C. 90%
   D. 95%

III. What is the specificity of the AI-assisted software in detecting AMD, in per cent and to the nearest whole number?
   A. 80%
   B. 82%
   C. 90%
   D. 95%

Optics 1

1. A.

The visible wavelengths of the electromagnetic spectrum fall between 400 nm and 780 nm.

Further reading

Chapter 1: Properties of light and visual function. In: Elkington AR, Frank HJ, Greaney MJ. *Clinical Optics*. Blackwell Science (1999).

2. C.

Radiant intensity is measured in watts per steradian and luminous intensity is measured in candelas, i.e. lumens per steradian. Other options are false.

Further reading

Chapter 1: Properties of light and visual function. In: Elkington AR, Frank HJ, Greaney MJ. *Clinical Optics*. Blackwell Science (1999).

3. C.

The image formed by the concave mirror where the object lies outside the centre of curvature is real, inverted, and diminished (RID). Fig. 1.1a–c displays three ray diagrams for images formed by a concave mirror, depending on the position of the object. Fig. 1.2 displays a ray diagram for the image formed by a convex mirror.

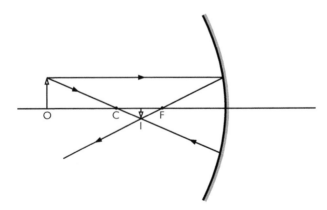

(a) O outside C; I = real, inverted, diminished (RID).

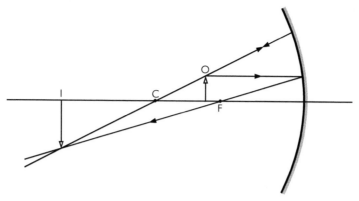

(b) O between C and F; I = real, inverted, and enlarged (RIE).

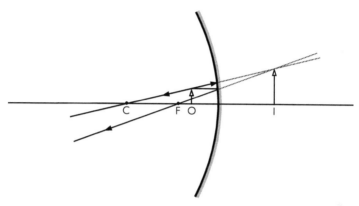

(c) O inside F; I = virtual, erect, and enlarged (VEE).

Figure 1.1 Image formation by concave mirror, where object is outside centre of curvature (a), between centre of curvature and principal focus (b), and inside principal focus (c). Key: O = object; I = image; C = centre of curvature; F = principal focus.

Figure courtesy of Mr Umar Ahmed, Medical Student, Imperial College London.

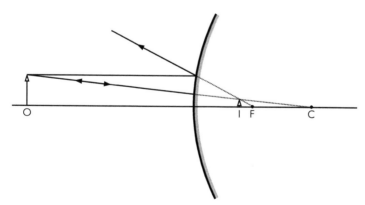

Figure 1.2 Image formation by convex mirror, where object at any distance from mirror. The image is virtual, erect, and diminished (VED).

Key: O = object; I = image; C = centre of curvature; F = principal focus.

Figure courtesy of Mr Umar Ahmed, Medical Student, Imperial College London.

Further reading

Chapter 2: Reflection of light. In: Elkington AR, Frank HJ, Greaney MJ. *Clinical Optics*. Blackwell Science (1999).

4. A.

Fibreoptic cables utilise total internal reflection.

Further reading

Chapter 3: Refraction of light. In: Elkington AR, Frank HJ, Greaney MJ. *Clinical Optics*. Blackwell Science (1999).

5. D.

The ×8 loupe possesses a lens power of 32 dioptres and is commonly used.

Further reading

Chapter 5: Spherical lenses. In: Elkington AR, Frank HJ, Greaney MJ. *Clinical Optics*. Blackwell Science (1999).

6. C.

Simple transposition of cylinders:

Step 1. Sum. Add the powers of sphere and cylinder to arrive at new power of sphere.

Step 2. Sign. Switch the sign of cylinder.

Step 3. Axis. Rotate axis of cylinder through 90°.

Further reading

Chapter 7: Optical prescriptions, spectacle lenses. In: Elkington AR, Frank HJ, Greaney MJ. *Clinical Optics*. Blackwell Science (1999).

7. C.

Fig. 1.3 displays Gullstrand's schematic eye and Table 1.1 displays distances behind the anterior corneal surface for Gullstrand's schematic eye. Table 1.2 displays refractive indices of the eye. Fig. 1.4 displays the reduced eye and Table 1.3 displays distances behind the anterior corneal surface for the reduced eye.

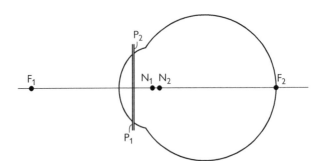

Figure 1.3 Gullstrand's schematic eye. Key: P_1 = first principal point; P_2 = second principal point; N_1 = first nodal point; N_2 = second nodal point; F_1 = first focal point; F_2 = second focal point.

Figure courtesy of Mr Umar Ahmed, Medical Student, Imperial College London.

Table 1.1 Distances of cardinal points behind the anterior corneal surface as per Gullstrand's schematic eye. Total refractive power: +58.64 dioptres

Cardinal points	Distance behind anterior corneal surface (mm)
P_1	1.35
P_2	1.60
N_1	7.08
N_2	7.33
F_1	−15.7
F_2	24.4

Key: P_1 = first principal point; P_2 = second principal point; N_1 = first nodal point; N_2 = second nodal point; F_1 = first focal point; F_2 = second focal point.

Table 1.2 Refractive indices of the eye

Refracting body	Refractive index
Air	1.000
Cornea	1.376
Aqueous humour	1.336
Lens (cortex–core)	1.386–1.406
Vitreous humour	1.336

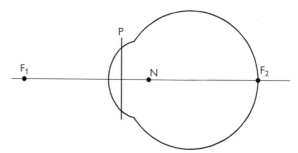

Figure 1.4 Reduced eye. Key: P = principal point; N = nodal point; F_1 = first focal point; F_2 = second focal point.

Figure courtesy of Mr Umar Ahmed, Medical Student, Imperial College London.

Table 1.3 Distances of cardinal points behind the anterior corneal surface as per the reduced eye. Total refractive power: +58.6 dioptres

Cardinal point	Distance behind anterior corneal surface (mm)
P	1.35
N	7.08
F_1	−15.7
F_2	24.13

Key: P = principal point; N = nodal point; F_1 = first focal point; F_2 = second focal point.

Further reading

Chapter 9: Refraction by the eye. In: Elkington AR, Frank HJ, Greaney MJ. *Clinical Optics*. Blackwell Science (1999).

8. A.

Manifest hypermetropia is defined as the strongest convex lens correction accepted for clear distance vision.

Further reading

Chapter 10: Optics of ametropia. In: Elkington AR, Frank HJ, Greaney MJ. *Clinical Optics*. Blackwell Science (1999).

9. D.

Barrel distortion can occur with high-powered concave lenses, whereas pin cushion distortion can occur with high-powered convex lenses.

Further reading

Chapter 10: Optics of ametropia. In: Elkington AR, Frank HJ, Greaney MJ. *Clinical Optics*. Blackwell Science (1999).

10. B.

In bifocals, prismatic jump can be minimised if the optical centres of the two lenses lie at or near to the junction of the distance and near portions.

Further reading

Chapter 11: Presbyopia. In: Elkington AR, Frank HJ, Greaney MJ. *Clinical Optics*. Blackwell Science (1999).

11. B.

The dark-adaptation stage relates to electroretinography, not retinoscopy. Retinoscopy aims to obtain an objective measurement of the refractive state of the eye.

Further reading

Chapter 14: Instruments. In: Elkington AR, Frank HJ, Greaney MJ. *Clinical Optics*. Blackwell Science (1999).

12. D.

The Javal–Schiøtz keratometer uses an object of variable size, consisting of a pair of mires (A and B), which each consist of a small lantern with a coloured window. Doubling of the image is achieved using a Wollaston prism.

Further reading

Chapter 14: Instruments. In: Elkington AR, Frank HJ, Greaney MJ. *Clinical Optics*. Blackwell Science (1999).

13. D.

The Hruby lens is a powerful plano-concave lens. The 90-dioptre lens provides a wider field of view but less magnification as compared to the 78-dioptre lens. The panfunduscope contact lens forms a real, inverted image of the fundus.

Further reading

Chapter 14: Instruments. In: Elkington AR, Frank HJ, Greaney MJ. *Clinical Optics*. Blackwell Science (1999).

14. D.

The acronym 'LASER' stands for the instrument's mode of action: Light Amplification by Stimulated Emission of Radiation.

Further reading

Chapter 15: Lasers. In: Elkington AR, Frank HJ, Greaney MJ. *Clinical Optics*. Blackwell Science (1999).

15. D.

Auto-refractors generally do not perform well if the ocular media are not clear, or in eyes with small or distorted pupils.

Further reading

Chapter 14: Instruments. In: Elkington AR, Frank HJ, Greaney MJ. *Clinical Optics*. Blackwell Science (1999).

16. A.

Blue and green light is scattered more than red light, because red light is of a longer wavelength. As the visibility of the vitreous depends on the scattering of the incident light, this makes blue and green (red-free) filters useful for inspecting the vitreous.

Further reading

Chapter 14: Instruments. In: Elkington AR, Frank HJ, Greaney MJ. *Clinical Optics*. Blackwell Science (1999).

Anatomy 1

17. B.

There are seven bones of the orbit: **M**axilla, **F**rontal, **Z**ygomatic, **E**thmoid, **L**acrimal, **S**phenoid, and **P**alatine. You can remember these with the following mnemonic: '**M**any **F**riendly **Z**ebras **E**njoy **L**azy **S**ummer **P**icnics'. Table 1.4 summarises the bony structures of the orbital walls.

Table 1.4 Bony structures of the orbital walls

Wall	Bony structures
Roof	Orbital plate of frontal bone and lesser wing of sphenoid
Floor	Orbital plate of maxilla, orbital surface of zygomatic, and orbital process of palatine
Lateral	Zygomatic bone and greater wing of sphenoid
Medial	Frontal process of maxilla, lacrimal bone, orbital plate of ethmoid, and body of sphenoid

Further reading

Chapter 1: Anatomy of the eye and orbit. In: Forrester JV, Dick AD, McMenamin PG, Roberts F, Pearlman E. *The Eye: Basic Sciences in Practice* (4th Edition). Elsevier (2016).

Chapter 3: The orbital cavity. In: Snell RS, Lemp MA. *Clinical Anatomy of the Eye* (2nd Edition). John Wiley and Sons (1998).

18. C.

When the eye is closed, the upper eyelid normally covers the entire cornea. The lower eyelid normally sits just below the cornea when the eye is open and only rises slightly on closure. Other responses are true.

Further reading

Chapter 5: The ocular appendages. In: Snell RS, Lemp MA. *Clinical Anatomy of the Eye* (2nd Edition). John Wiley and Sons (1998).

19. C.

The fibres of the palpebral portion sweep concentrically and laterally across the lids, in front of the orbital septum. The lacrimal portion also helps to dilate the lacrimal sac during blinking, which sucks tears from the lacus lacrimalis into the lacrimal punctum.

Further reading

Chapter 1: Anatomy of the eye and orbit. In: Forrester JV, Dick AD, McMenamin PG, Roberts F, Pearlman E. *The Eye: Basic Sciences in Practice* (4th Edition). Elsevier (2016).

Chapter 5: The ocular appendages. In: Snell RS, Lemp MA. *Clinical Anatomy of the Eye* (2nd Edition). John Wiley and Sons (1998).

20. C.

The following nerves pass through the common tendinous ring (also known as the annulus of Zinn): upper division of oculomotor, nasociliary, abducent, and lower division of oculomotor. The medial aspect of the common tendinous ring also contains the optical canal, through which the optic nerve and ophthalmic artery pass. Fig. 1.5 is an anatomical illustration of the superior orbital fissure and common tendinous ring.

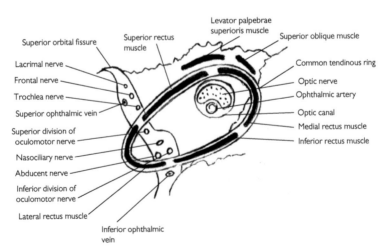

Figure 1.5 The superior orbital fissure and common tendinous ring (right orbit).

Figure courtesy of Mr Syed Riyaz Ahmad, retired ophthalmologist, Essex, UK.

Further reading

Chapter 1: Anatomy of the eye and orbit. In: Forrester JV, Dick AD, McMenamin PG, Roberts F, Pearlman E. *The Eye: Basic Sciences in Practice* (4th Edition). Elsevier (2016).

Chapter 3: The orbital cavity. In: Snell RS, Lemp MA. *Clinical Anatomy of the Eye* (2nd Edition). John Wiley and Sons (1998).

21. A.

The sclera is known as the lamina cribrosa at the site where it is pierced by the optic nerve.

Further reading

Chapter 6: The eyeball. In: Snell RS, Lemp MA. *Clinical Anatomy of the Eye* (2nd Edition). John Wiley and Sons (1998).

22. B.

The peripheral cornea is supplied with oxygen by diffusion from the anterior ciliary blood vessels. Other responses are true.

Further reading

Chapter 6: The eyeball. In: Snell RS, Lemp MA. *Clinical Anatomy of the Eye* (2nd Edition). John Wiley and Sons (1998).

23. D.

The pituitary fossa is an indentation in the roof of the body of sphenoid. It is anteriorly bound by the tuberculum sellae and posteriorly bound by the dorsum sellae.

Further reading

Chapter 1: Anatomy of the eye and orbit. In: Forrester JV, Dick AD, McMenamin PG, Roberts F, Pearlman E. *The Eye: Basic Sciences in Practice* (4th Edition). Elsevier (2016).

24. C.

Fig. 1.6 displays the layers of the retina as seen on optical coherence tomography. The correct order of the layers of the retina, from inner (closest to the vitreous) to outer (closest to the choroid), is as follows: **I**nternal limiting membrane, **N**erve fibre layer, **G**anglion cell layer, **I**nner plexiform layer,

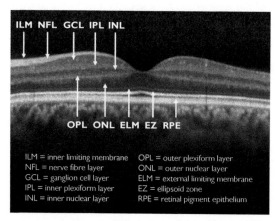

Figure 1.6 Layers of the retina.

Figure courtesy of Dr Sohaib Rufai. © Sohaib R. Rufai 2021.

Inner nuclear layer, Outer plexiform layer, Outer nuclear layer, External limiting membrane, Ellipsoid zone, Retinal pigment epithelium. A helpful mnemonic to remember this is as follows: In New Generation, It Isn't Only Ophthalmologists Examining Every Retina.

Further reading

Chapter 6: The eyeball. In: Snell RS, Lemp MA. *Clinical Anatomy of the Eye* (2nd Edition). John Wiley and Sons (1998).

25. C.

The four parts of the optic nerve have the following approximate lengths: intraocular, 1 mm; intraorbital, 25 mm; intracanalicular, 5 mm; intracranial, 10 mm.

Further reading

Chapter 13: The visual pathway. In: Snell RS, Lemp MA. *Clinical Anatomy of the Eye* (2nd Edition). John Wiley and Sons (1998).

26. C.

The correct order of structures of the anterior chamber angle as seen on gonioscopy, from posterior to anterior, is as follows: Iris, Ciliary body, Scleral spur, Trabecular meshwork, Schwalbe's line. An easy way to remember this is using the following mnemonic: I Can't See This Stuff.

Further reading

Chapter 7: The anatomy of the eyeball as seen with the ophthalmoscope, slit lamp and gonioscope. In: Snell RS, Lemp MA. *Clinical Anatomy of the Eye* (2nd Edition). John Wiley and Sons (1998).

27. D.

Type A muscle fibres are responsible for saccadic eye movements, while type B muscle fibres are required for smooth pursuit. Other options are true.

Further reading

Chapter 1: Anatomy of the eye and orbit. In: Forrester JV, Dick AD, McMenamin PG, Roberts F, Pearlman E. *The Eye: Basic Sciences in Practice* (4th Edition). Elsevier (2016).

28. C.

The secondary action of the superior oblique is abduction. Table 1.5 summarises the innervation and actions of the extraocular muscles.

Table 1.5 Innervation and actions of the extraocular muscles

Muscle	Innervation	Primary action	Secondary action	Tertiary action
Superior rectus	Oculomotor (superior division)	Elevation	Adduction	Intorsion
Inferior rectus	Oculomotor (inferior division)	Depression	Adduction	Extorsion
Medial rectus	Oculomotor (inferior division)	Adduction	None	None
Lateral rectus	Abducens	Abduction	None	None
Superior oblique	Trochlear	Depression	Abduction	Intorsion
Inferior oblique	Oculomotor (inferior division)	Elevation	Abduction	Extorsion

Further reading

Chapter 8: Movements of the eyeball and the extraocular muscles. In: Snell RS, Lemp MA. *Clinical Anatomy of the Eye* (2nd Edition). John Wiley and Sons (1998).

29. C.

The ipsilateral eye sends visual information to layers 2, 3, and 5 of the lateral geniculate nucleus, whereas the contralateral eye sends information to layers 1, 4, and 6.

Further reading

Chapter 13: The visual pathway. In: Snell RS, Lemp MA. *Clinical Anatomy of the Eye* (2nd Edition). John Wiley and Sons (1998).

30. A.

The lens placode can be identified on day 27 of embryological development (Forrester et al., 2016). Please note that the Snell textbook (1998) states 22 days.

Further reading

Chapter 1: Anatomy of the eye and orbit. In: Forrester JV, Dick AD, McMenamin PG, Roberts F, Pearlman E. *The Eye: Basic Sciences in Practice* (4th Edition). Elsevier (2016).

Physiology 1

Physiology of the eye and vision

31. A.

Optical coherence tomography has demonstrated that the precorneal tear film is 3.4 micrometres (± 2.6 micrometres).

Further reading

Dartt DA. Chapter 15: Formation and function of the tear film. In: Levin LA, Nilsson SFE, Ver Hoeve J, et al. *Adler's Physiology of the Eye* (11th Edition). Elsevier (2011).

32. C.

The unconventional outflow pathway of aqueous humour at the anterior chamber angle is also known as the uveoscleral or posterior route. Option B represents the conventional outflow pathway, also known as the trabecular route.

Further reading

Gabelt BT, Kaufman PL. Chapter 11: Production and flow of aqueous humor. In: Levin LA, Nilsson SFE, Ver Hoeve J, et al. *Adler's Physiology of the Eye* (11th Edition). Elsevier (2011).

33. C.

The elongated lens fibres converge at three planes, forming a 'Y'-shaped suture anteriorly and inverted 'Y' posteriorly.

Further reading

Beebe DC. Chapter 5: The lens. In: Levin LA, Nilsson SFE, Ver Hoeve J, et al. *Adler's Physiology of the Eye* (11th Edition). Elsevier (2011).

34. A.

The resting membrane potential of a dark-adapted rod cell is approximately −40 mV.

Further reading

Gross AK, Wensel TG. Chapter 18: Biochemical cascade of phototransduction. In: Levin LA, Nilsson SFE, Ver Hoeve J, et al. *Adler's Physiology of the Eye* (11th Edition). Elsevier (2011).

35. B.

Bloch's law assumes a monotonic increase in perceived contrast with increased duration, as the law states that the intensity of the threshold stimulus is inversely proportional to its duration.

Further reading

Chapter 5: Physiology of vision and the visual system. In: Forrester JV, Dick AD, McMenamin PG, Roberts F, Pearlman E. *The Eye: Basic Sciences in Practice* (4th Edition). Elsevier (2016).

36. C.

The pupillary light reflex aims to maintain constant retinal illumination in response to changes in lighting. Pupil input from retinal ganglion cells leaves the optic tract in the brachium of the superior colliculus. Postganglionic parasympathetic neurons pass from the ciliary ganglion via the short ciliary nerves to the iris sphincter muscle.

Further reading

Kardon R. Chapter 25: Regulation of light through the pupil. In: Levin LA, Nilsson SFE, Ver Hoeve J, et al. *Adler's Physiology of the Eye* (11th Edition). Elsevier (2011).

37. D.

OPN1MW: middle-wavelength sensitive cone opsin, expressed in M cones (aka 'green' cones); absence of this gene is most commonly associated with deutan defects. *OPN1LW*: long-wavelength sensitive cone opsin, expressed in L cones (aka 'red' cones); absence of this gene is most commonly associated with protan defects. *OPN1SW*: short-wavelength sensitive cone opsin, expressed in S cones (aka 'blue' cones); tritan defects are caused by a missense mutation in one copy of this gene. *OPN1DW* is a fictional 'distractor' and not the name of any known gene.

Further reading

Neitz J, Mancuso K, Kuchenbecker JA, Neitz M. Chapter 34: Color vision. In: Levin LA, Nilsson SFE, Ver Hoeve J, et al. *Adler's Physiology of the Eye* (11th Edition). Elsevier (2011).

General physiology

38. B.

The action potential can be summarised in three stages: resting stage, depolarisation stage, and repolarisation stage. There is a negative membrane potential (−90 millivolts) present during the resting stage. During depolarisation, the nerve fibre membrane becomes permeable to sodium ions, permitting a huge number to diffuse inside the axon. In larger nerve fibres, an excess of positive sodium ions can cause the membrane to 'overshoot' above the zero level during depolarisation.

In some smaller fibres and many neurons of the central nervous system, the potential approaches the zero level without overshooting. During repolarisation, the sodium channels close and the potassium channels open to a greater degree than normal, thus re-establishing the normal negative resting membrane potential. Fig. 1.7 summarises the stages of the action potential.

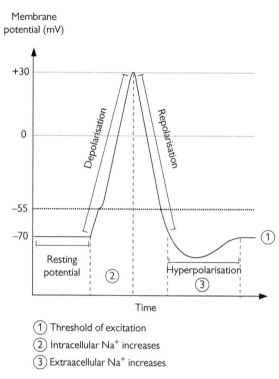

① Threshold of excitation
② Intracellular Na$^+$ increases
③ Extraacellular Na$^+$ increases

Figure 1.7 The action potential. Key: Na$^+$ = sodium ions.

Figure courtesy of Mr Umar Ahmed, Medical Student, Imperial College London.

Further reading

Chapter 5: Membrane potentials and action potentials. In: Hall JE. *Guyton and Hall Textbook of Medical Physiology* (13th Edition). Elsevier (2016).

39. D.

Tachycardia is defined as a heart rate faster than 100 beats per minute. First-degree AV block is characterised by a prolonged PR interval greater than 0.20 seconds. Second-degree type I AV block (Wenckebach periodicity) is characterised by a progressive prolongation of the PR interval until a ventricular beat is skipped. Second-degree type II AV block typically features a fixed number of non-conducted P waves per QRS complex (e.g. 2:1 block). In third-degree AV block (complete AV block), the P waves are dissociated from the QRS–T complexes.

Further reading

Chapter 13: Cardiac arrhythmias and their electrocardiographic interpretation. In: Hall JE. *Guyton and Hall Textbook of Medical Physiology* (13th Edition). Elsevier (2016).

40. C.

It is the opening of ion channels that causes receptor potentials, not their closure. Receptor potentials can be caused by four mechanisms applied to the receptor: mechanical deformation, application of a chemical, change in temperature, and effects of electromagnetic radiation.

Further reading

Chapter 47: Sensory receptors, neuronal circuits for processing information. In: Hall JE. *Guyton and Hall Textbook of Medical Physiology* (13th Edition). Elsevier (2016).

41. B.

The anterior pituitary gland secretes **F**ollicle-stimulating hormone (FSH), **L**uteinising hormone (LH), **A**drenocorticotropic hormone (ACTH), **T**hyroid-stimulating hormone (TSH), **P**rolactin, **E**ndorphins, and **G**rowth hormone (GH). These can be remembered using the mnemonic, **FLAT PEG**. The posterior pituitary gland secretes antidiuretic hormone and oxytocin.

Further reading

Chapter 75: Introduction to endocrinology. In: Hall JE. *Guyton and Hall Textbook of Medical Physiology* (13th Edition). Elsevier (2016).

Biochemistry

42. B.

Chromatin is the main nuclear component and consists of highly extended DNA, RNA, and protein in the interphase cell (non-dividing). It becomes significantly condensed by 400-fold during cell division to form chromosomes. Chromatin packing results from interaction between negatively charged DNA and histones, which, at the pH of the cell, carry a positive charge. Euchromatin is less packed than heterochromatin.

Further reading

Chapter 4: Biochemistry and cell biology. In: Forrester JV, Dick AD, McMenamin PG, Roberts F, Pearlman E. *The Eye: Basic Sciences in Practice* (5th Edition). Elsevier (2021).

43. B.

The central vitreous body possesses a lower concentration of hyaluronan and collagen as compared to the cortex. In addition, while hyaluronan is the sole glycosaminoglycan (GAG) found in the central vitreous gel, the cortex contains other GAGs including chondroitin sulphate (3.5%) and heparan sulphate (0.3%). These may be important in vitreo/retinal apposition.

Further reading

Chapter 4: Biochemistry and cell biology. In: Forrester JV, Dick AD, McMenamin PG, Roberts F, Pearlman E. *The Eye: Basic Sciences in Practice* (5th Edition). Elsevier (2021).

Pathology 1

General and ocular pathology

44. B.

Following transendothelial migration and extravasation, the movement of leucocytes is subsequently controlled by chemotaxis. Phagocytosis involves opsonisation of bacteria by complement components followed by engulfment within leucocytes. Histamine and leukotrienes increase vascular permeability.

Further reading

Chapter 9: Pathology. In: Forrester JV, Dick AD, McMenamin PG, Roberts F, Pearlman E. *The Eye: Basic Sciences in Practice* (4th Edition). Elsevier (2016).

45. B.

Scar tissue in the sclera is derived from episcleral fibroblasts, whereas that in the choroid is derived from scleral fibroblasts.

Further reading

Chapter 9: Pathology. In: Forrester JV, Dick AD, McMenamin PG, Roberts F, Pearlman E. *The Eye: Basic Sciences in Practice* (4th Edition). Elsevier (2016).

46. C.

In cataractogenesis, accumulation of yellow pigments causes increased absorption of blue light.

Further reading

Chapter 9: Pathology. In: Forrester JV, Dick AD, McMenamin PG, Roberts F, Pearlman E. *The Eye: Basic Sciences in Practice* (4th Edition). Elsevier (2016).

47. D.

In Sjögren's syndrome, there is a loss of goblet cells in the conjunctival epithelium and squamous metaplasia of the surface epithelium.

Further reading

Chapter 9: Pathology. In: Forrester JV, Dick AD, McMenamin PG, Roberts F, Pearlman E. *The Eye: Basic Sciences in Practice* (4th Edition). Elsevier (2016).

48. D.

In vitelliform dystrophy (Best disease), there is an accumulation of lipofuscin in the retinal pigment epithelium and atrophy of the photoreceptor layer.

Further reading

Chapter 9: Pathology. In: Forrester JV, Dick AD, McMenamin PG, Roberts F, Pearlman E. *The Eye: Basic Sciences in Practice* (4th Edition). Elsevier (2016).

49. C.

The following mnemonic can help you remember common corneal stains: **M**arilyn **M**onroe **A**lways **G**ets **H**er **M**akeup in **LA** **C**ity. Table 1.6 summarises these three stains used for the histopathological diagnosis of stromal corneal dystrophies. Fig. 1.8 displays histopathological slides for lattice, granular, and macular dystrophy.

Table 1.6 Stains used for histopathalogical diagnosis of stromal corneal dystrophies

Corneal dystrophy	Component	Stain
Macular	Mucopolysaccharide	Alcian blue
Granular	Hyaline	Masson trichrome
Lattice	Amyloid	Congo red

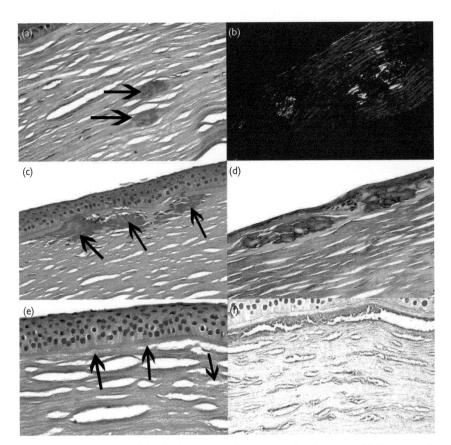

Figure 1.8 Histopathological slides for lattice, granular, and macular dystrophy. (a) Haematoxylin and eosin (H&E)-stained section of cornea showing spindle-shaped eosinophilic amyloid deposits (arrows) in the corneal stroma typical of lattice dystrophy. (b) Congo red staining of the section in part (a) viewed under polarised light, showing green birefringence of the amyloid deposits. (c) H&E-stained section of cornea showing irregular, eosinophilic, hyaline-like deposits (arrows) in the anterior stroma associated with Bowman's layer effacement, typical of granular dystrophy. (d) Masson trichrome staining of the section in part (c) showing the crimson staining of the hyaline-like deposits of granular dystrophy and blue staining of the stromal collagen fibres. (e) H&E-stained section of cornea showing greyish granular deposits beneath Bowman's layer and between the stromal collagen (arrows) of macular dystrophy. (f) Alcian blue staining of the section in part (e) showing grain-like blue staining of the macular dystrophy deposits beneath Bowman's layer and between the stromal collagen fibres.

Figure courtesy of Dr Hardeep Singh Mudhar, Consultant Ophthalmic Pathologist, Royal Hallamshire Hospital.

Further reading

Chapter 9: Pathology. In: Forrester JV, Dick AD, McMenamin PG, Roberts F, Pearlman E. *The Eye: Basic Sciences in Practice* (4th Edition). Elsevier (2016).

50. C.

Type 1 herpes simplex virus can cause dendritic ulceration within the corneal epithelium. Primary infection often occurs through the oral mucosa, as well as the lips and facial skin. When reactivated, the virus travels along the sensory nerves to the corneal epithelium. Option D is applicable to herpes zoster ophthalmicus.

Further reading

Chapter 9: Pathology. In: Forrester JV, Dick AD, McMenamin PG, Roberts F, Pearlman E. *The Eye: Basic Sciences in Practice* (4th Edition). Elsevier (2016).

51. B.

The most common primary sites for choroidal metastasis are breast, prostate, lung, and gastrointestinal tract.

Further reading

Chapter 9: Pathology. In: Forrester JV, Dick AD, McMenamin PG, Roberts F, Pearlman E. *The Eye: Basic Sciences in Practice* (4th Edition). Elsevier (2016).

Microbiology

52. B.

Neutrophils make up approximately 25% of total white cells in normal individuals, representing the blood's most abundant leucocytes.

Further reading

Chapter 8: Microbial infections of the eye. In: Forrester JV, Dick AD, McMenamin PG, Roberts F, Pearlman E. *The Eye: Basic Sciences in Practice* (4th Edition). Elsevier (2016).

53. A.

Staphylococcus epidermidis is the most common cause of postoperative pseudophakic endophthalmitis (i.e. following cataract surgery).

Further reading

Chapter 8: Microbial infections of the eye. In: Forrester JV, Dick AD, McMenamin PG, Roberts F, Pearlman E. *The Eye: Basic Sciences in Practice* (4th Edition). Elsevier (2016).

54. B.

Both *Toxocara canis* and *Toxocara cati* are nematodes. They are transmitted by dogs and cats, respectively. Trematodes and cestodes are parasitic flatworms (platyhelminths). Protozoans are single-celled eukaryotes (e.g. *Acanthamoeba*).

Further reading

Chapter 8: Microbial infections of the eye. In: Forrester JV, Dick AD, McMenamin PG, Roberts F, Pearlman E. *The Eye: Basic Sciences in Practice* (4th Edition). Elsevier (2016).

Immunology

55. A.

The mononuclear phagocyte system includes monocytes, macrophages, and dendritic cells. The granulocyte series of cells include mast cells, basophils, and eosinophils.

Further reading

Chapter 7: Immunology. In: Forrester JV, Dick AD, McMenamin PG, Roberts F, Pearlman E. *The Eye: Basic Sciences in Practice* (4th Edition). Elsevier (2016).

56. B.

HLA-B27 is associated with ankylosing spondylitis. HLA-A29 is associated with birdshot retinochoroidopathy. HLA-B51 is associated with Behçet's retinal vasculitis.

Further reading

Chapter 7: Immunology. In: Forrester JV, Dick AD, McMenamin PG, Roberts F, Pearlman E. *The Eye: Basic Sciences in Practice* (4th Edition). Elsevier (2016).

Pharmacology and genetics 1

Pharmacology

57. A.

Fick's law of diffusion states that drugs cross a cell membrane at a rate directly proportional to the concentration gradient across the membrane and the diffusion coefficient, and inversely proportional to the membrane thickness. Sherrington's law of reciprocal innervation explains that a muscle will relax when its opposite muscle contracts. The Frank–Starling law of the heart postulates that the force developed in a muscle fibre is dependent on how much the fibre is stretched. Poiseuille's law states that the flow of fluid through a tube (e.g. blood vessel) is related to the viscosity of the fluid (blood), the pressure gradient across the tube (vessel), and the length and diameter of the tube (vessel).

Further reading

Chapter 6: General and ocular pharmacology. In: Forrester JV, Dick AD, McMenamin PG, Roberts F, Pearlman E. *The Eye: Basic Sciences in Practice* (5th Edition). Elsevier (2021).

58. B.

The approximate natural tear volume is 7–8 μL. This is relevant for the topical administration of ocular drugs.

Further reading

Chapter 6: General and ocular pharmacology. In: Forrester JV, Dick AD, McMenamin PG, Roberts F, Pearlman E. *The Eye: Basic Sciences in Practice* (5th Edition). Elsevier (2021).

59. B.

Phenylephrine is a non-selective an α-agonist. Apraclonidine is an α_2 partial agonist. Brimonidine is a selective α_2-agonist. Cocaine inhibits the uptake of noradrenaline at nerve endings.

Further reading

Chapter 6: General and ocular pharmacology. In: Forrester JV, Dick AD, McMenamin PG, Roberts F, Pearlman E. *The Eye: Basic Sciences in Practice* (5th Edition). Elsevier (2021).

60. A.

The pH of local anaesthetic is **altered** with the addition of adrenaline solution (acidic). Local anaesthetics comprise an **aromatic residue** linked to an amide or basic side chain; the aromatic residue is hydrophobic and the amide group hydrophilic.

Further reading

Chapter 6: General and ocular pharmacology. In: Forrester JV, Dick AD, McMenamin PG, Roberts F, Pearlman E. *The Eye: Basic Sciences in Practice* (5th Edition). Elsevier (2021).

61. B.

Infliximab is a chimeric monoclonal antibody.

Further reading

Chapter 6: General and ocular pharmacology. In: Forrester JV, Dick AD, McMenamin PG, Roberts F, Pearlman E. *The Eye: Basic Sciences in Practice* (5th Edition). Elsevier (2021).

62. A.

Brimonidine is a selective α_2-receptor agonist. It is used to lower intraocular pressure.

Further reading

Chapter 6: General and ocular pharmacology. In: Forrester JV, Dick AD, McMenamin PG, Roberts F, Pearlman E. *The Eye: Basic Sciences in Practice* (5th Edition). Elsevier (2021).

Genetics

63. D.

The stages of mitosis are correctly ordered and summarised as follows:

1. Prophase—chromosomes condense.
2. Metaphase—chromosomes align in the centre of the nucleus.
3. Anaphase—centromere of the chromosomes divides with chromatid separation.
4. Telophase—daughter chromosomes separate.

These stages can be remembered using the acronym, **PMAT**.

Further reading

Chapter 3: Genetics. In: Forrester JV, Dick AD, McMenamin PG, Roberts F, Pearlman E. *The Eye: Basic Sciences in Practice* (5th Edition). Elsevier (2021).

64. D.

Patau syndrome is associated with trisomy 13. Klinefelter syndrome (47, XXY) occurs when a male has an additional X chromosome. Down syndrome is associated with trisomy 21.

Further reading

Chapter 3: Genetics. In: Forrester JV, Dick AD, McMenamin PG, Roberts F, Pearlman E. *The Eye: Basic Sciences in Practice* (5th Edition). Elsevier (2021).

65. C.

The acrosome of the sperm is lost during fertilisation, thus mitochondrial inheritance is exclusively maternal.

Further reading

Chapter 3: Genetics. In: Forrester JV, Dick AD, McMenamin PG, Roberts F, Pearlman E. *The Eye: Basic Sciences in Practice* (5th Edition). Elsevier (2021).

66. A.

PAX6 mutation is associated with aniridia. *RS1* mutation is associated with juvenile X-linked retinoschisis. *RB1* mutation is associated with retinoblastoma.

Further reading

Chapter 3: Genetics. In: Forrester JV, Dick AD, McMenamin PG, Roberts F, Pearlman E. *The Eye: Basic Sciences in Practice* (5th Edition). Elsevier (2021).

67. A.

Naked DNA can be injected using a gene gun, but this is an **inefficient** way to transfer DNA fragments.

Further reading

Chapter 3: Genetics. In: Forrester JV, Dick AD, McMenamin PG, Roberts F, Pearlman E. *The Eye: Basic Sciences in Practice* (5th Edition). Elsevier (2021).

68. B.

There are two approaches to identify abnormal genes among the millions of genes present in the human genome. One is to find a gene marker in the human genome close to the culprit gene defect—this is the basis of linkage analysis, not candidate gene analysis, which represents the other approach. Candidate gene analysis aims to identify genes specifically expressed, or those known to code for important proteins, in the tissue in question. Knowledge of the functions of proteins from the genes in question is not required, but can improve understanding of the underlying pathophysiology of the condition in question.

Further reading

Chapter 3: Genetics. In: Forrester JV, Dick AD, McMenamin PG, Roberts F, Pearlman E. *The Eye: Basic Sciences in Practice* (5th Edition). Elsevier (2021).

Investigations 1

69. B.

The Maddox rod test can be used to assess symptomatic phorias. The phoria can be quantified by neutralising prisms. A single Maddox rod (i.e. series of red cylinders) is positioned horizontally in front of the right eye fixing on a white spot of light. The line should pass through the spot if the patient has no horizontal phoria. If the line appears to the right of the white spot, the patient has right esophoria. If the line appears to the left of the white spot, the patient has right exophoria. The Maddox rod can be rotated vertically to identify vertical phorias.

Further reading

Denniston AKO, Wolffsohn J, Auld R, Murray PI. Chapter 1: Clinical skills. In: Denniston AKO, Murray PI. *Oxford Handbook of Ophthalmology*. Oxford University Press (2018).

70. A.

The cover test reveals manifest deviation, i.e. tropias. This deviation is always present. The patient is asked to fix on a target. If the left eye moves inwards upon covering the right eye, this indicates the left eye was previously divergent, i.e. left exotropia. Outward movement indicates esotropia. Downward movement indicates hypertropia. Upward movement indicates hypotropia. By contrast, the uncover test can reveal latent deviation, i.e. phorias.

Further reading

Denniston AKO, Wolffsohn J, Auld R, Murray PI. Chapter 1: Clinical Skills. In: Denniston AKO, Murray PI. *Oxford Handbook of Ophthalmology*. Oxford University Press (2018).

71. D.

Pie in the sky is most likely to be caused by a temporal lobe lesion and pie on the floor by a parietal lobe lesion. Central scotoma is most likely to be caused by macular lesions, optic neuritis, optic atrophy, and occipital cortex lesions.

Further reading

Mollan SP, Calcagni A, Keane PA. Chapter 2: Investigations and their interpretation. In: Denniston AKO, Murray PI. *Oxford Handbook of Ophthalmology*. Oxford University Press (2018).

72. C.

In keratometry, only the anterior surface of the **central cornea** (approximately 3 mm in diameter) is measured. It is typically expressed as 'k' values, which are two corneal curvature values, **90°** apart. Automated keratometry can be performed by **corneal topographers**, **autorefractors**, and the **IOLMaster®** (Zeiss)—the latter is used to provide intraocular lens (IOL) calculations for cataract surgery.

Further reading

Mollan SP, Calcagni A, Keane PA. Chapter 2: Investigations and their interpretation. In: Denniston AKO, Murray PI. *Oxford Handbook of Ophthalmology*. Oxford University Press (2018).

73. B.

Fluorescein allergy, renal impairment, and pregnancy are relative contraindications to fundus fluorescein angiography. Allergy to iodine or shellfish contraindicates indocyanine green angiography.

Further reading

Mollan SP, Calcagni A, Keane PA. Chapter 2: Investigations and their interpretation. In: Denniston AKO, Murray PI. *Oxford Handbook of Ophthalmology*. Oxford University Press (2018).

74. B.

Indocyanine green (ICG) is **98%** bound to serum proteins that do not pass through choriocapillaris vessel fenestrations. ICG absorbs and emits light in the near infrared range (absorption: approximately 810 nm; emission: approximately 830 nm). Window defect is commonly caused by retinal pigment epithelium defect. ICG angiography is **contraindicated** in pregnancy.

Further reading

Mollan SP, Calcagni A, Keane PA. Chapter 2: Investigations and their interpretation. In: Denniston AKO, Murray PI. *Oxford Handbook of Ophthalmology*. Oxford University Press (2018).

75. C.

OCTA is a non-invasive imaging modality that permits visualisation of the retinal and choroidal vasculature. Unlike fundus fluorescein angiography (FFA), it does not require an intravenous contrast agent. It delivers higher resolution and is much quicker to perform than FFA. However, recognition of artefact is important when performing OCTA, whereas FFA features less artefact.

Further reading

Mollan SP, Calcagni A, Keane PA. Chapter 2: Investigations and their interpretation. In: Denniston AKO, Murray PI. *Oxford Handbook of Ophthalmology*. Oxford University Press (2018).

76. D.

The axial resolution of ocular ultrasound is typically 150 μm and the transverse resolution is typically 450 μm.

Further reading

Mollan SP, Calcagni A, Keane PA. Chapter 2: Investigations and their interpretation. In: Denniston AKO, Murray PI. *Oxford Handbook of Ophthalmology*. Oxford University Press (2018).

77. C.

In applanation tonometry, intraocular pressure can be overestimated in patients with thick corneas and underestimated in those with thin corneas. Pachymetry can therefore help to estimate the accuracy of applanation tonometry.

Further reading

Mollan SP, Calcagni A, Keane PA. Chapter 2: Investigations and their interpretation. In: Denniston AKO, Murray PI. *Oxford Handbook of Ophthalmology*. Oxford University Press (2018).

78. C.

Please see Fig. 1.9 displaying the normal pattern electroretinogram and pattern VEP waveforms.

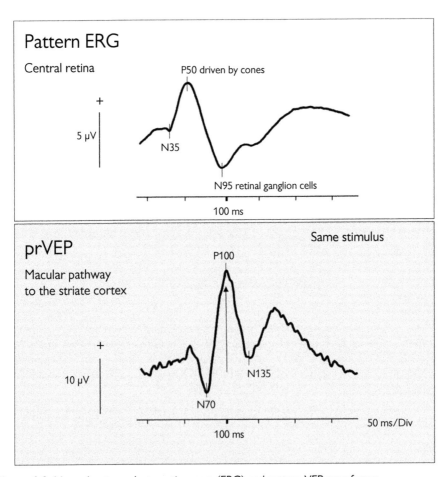

Figure 1.9 Normal pattern electroretinogram (ERG) and pattern VEP waveforms.
Courtesy of Dr Dorothy A. Thompson, Consultant Clinical Scientist, Great Ormond Street Hospital for Children.

Further reading

Mollan SP, Calcagni A, Keane PA. Chapter 2: Investigations and their interpretation. In: Denniston AKO, Murray PI. *Oxford Handbook of Ophthalmology*. Oxford University Press (2018).

79. C.

The VEP measures visual cortex activity in response to one of the following: i) pattern reversal, using a reversing black-and-white chequerboard (prVEP); ii) pattern onset/offset, where a chequerboard is abruptly exchanged with a grey background; iii) a flashing light (flash VEP). The pattern VEP reflects the central macular visual field and macular pathway function. The prVEP has most consistent timing and waveform shape among individuals. The flash VEP waveform varies most between individuals, but it is useful for inter-ocular comparison and for patients with limited cooperation such as young infants. The prVEP is characterised by a negative deflection at 75 milliseconds (N75), followed by a positive deflection at 100 milliseconds (P100), followed by another negative deflection at 135 milliseconds (N135). In albinism, trans-occipital crossed asymmetry can occur where the VEP is largest on one hemisphere for the right eye and the other hemisphere for the left eye.

Further reading

Handley SE, Šuštar M, Tekavčič Pompe M. What can visual electrophysiology tell about possible visual-field defects in paediatric patients. *Eye (Lond)*. 2021 Sep;35(9):2354–2373.

Odom JV, Bach M, Brigell M, et al. ISCEV standard for clinical visual evoked potentials: (2016 update). *Documenta Ophthalmologica. Advances in Ophthalmology*. 2016 Aug;133(1):1–9.

Miscellaneous 1

80. B.

In hypothesis testing, the p-value is the probability of obtaining the observed data or data that were more extreme due to chance if the null hypothesis (H_0) were true. The significance level (α) is conventionally set to 5%. A type I error (false positive) occurs when the null hypothesis (H_0) is incorrectly rejected, whereas a type II error (false negative) occurs where H_0 is incorrectly accepted. Power = $1 - \beta$ where β is the probability of a type II error. A power of 80% or greater is generally considered acceptable in study design, although many investigators would aim for higher than this.

Further reading

Bunce C, Patel KV, Xing W, et al. Ophthalmic statistics note 2: absence of evidence is not evidence of absence. *British Journal of Ophthalmology*. 2014;98(5):703–705.

81. D.

CONSORT = Consolidated Standards of Reporting Randomised Trials. STROBE = Strengthening the Reporting of Observational Studies in Epidemiology. STARD = Standards for Reporting of Diagnostic accuracy studies. PRISMA = Preferred Reporting Items for Systematic Reviews and

Meta-Analyses. See the EQUATOR Network website for other reporting guidelines with full details.

Further reading

EQUATOR Network. Enhancing the Quality and Transparency of Health Research. Available at: https://www.equator-network.org Accessed October 2021.

82. B.

Data can be classified as **quantitative** or **categorical**. **Quantitative** data are obtained by measurement and can be subclassified as continuous (lying on a continuum, e.g. height in cm, weight in kg) or as discrete (can only take certain values, e.g. number of patients). Data that are not obtained by measurement are termed **categorical**. If only two possible categories exist (e.g. dead or alive) this is subclassified as **binary** (or dichotomous). If the data can be placed in order (e.g. A-level grades) they are termed **ordinal**. If the data cannot be placed in order (e.g. eye colour), they are termed **nominal**. A common example of ordinal data is the **Likert scale**, a psychometric rating scale often used in surveys. For example, 'strongly agree; agree; neither agree nor disagree; disagree; strongly disagree'.

Further reading

Bunce C, Young-Zvandasara T. Simplified Ophthalmic Statistics (SOS). Part 1: an introduction to data—how do we classify it and why does it matter? *Eye News*. 2018;24(6):36–37. Available at: https://www.eyenews.uk.com/professional-development/trainees/post/simplified-ophthalmic-sta tistics-sos-part-1-an-introduction-to-data-how-do-we-classify-it-and-why-does-it-matter Accessed October 2021.

Denniston AKO, Moseley M, Murray PI. Chapter 26: Evidence-based ophthalmology. In: Denniston AKO, Murray PI. *Oxford Handbook of Ophthalmology*. Oxford University Press (2018).

83. B.

The **mean** value is the 'average' value, which can be calculated by adding all the data points then dividing by the number of data points. The **median** value is the 'middle' value, which can be found using the following method: (i) order the data points from smallest to largest; (ii) add 1 to the total number of data points then halve this number; (iii) if the result is a whole number, such as 3, then the median value is the 3rd number, whereas if the result is a decimal number, such as 5.5, then the median value lies halfway between the 5th and 6th number (i.e. the average of these two numbers). The **mode** is the most frequently occurring number. This can be easier to identify after ordering the numbers from smallest to largest. In this example:

31, 34, 34, 40, 48, 48, 48, 52, 54, 54, 60

The mode is 48 as this data point occurs the most frequently (three times).

Further reading

Bunce C, Young-Zvandasara T. Simplified Ophthalmic Statistics (SOS). Part 2: how to summarise your data and why it's a good idea to do so. *Eye News*. 2018;25(2):34–35. Available at: https://www.eyen ews.uk.com/education/trainees/post/sos-simplified-ophthalmic-statistics-part-2-how-to-summarise- your-data-and-why-it-s-a-good-idea-to-do-so Accessed October 2021.

84. B.

When the outcome measure is continuous (intraocular pressure) and the data parametric, use the unpaired *t*-test for unpaired data, as in this example. Fig. 1.10 is a flowchart displaying common statistical tests and rules.

Further reading

Bunce C, Young-Zvandasara T. Simplified Ophthalmic Statistics (SOS). Part 3: which statistical test should I use (if any)? *Eye News.* 2019;25(4):34–36. Available at: https://www.eyenews.uk.com/educat ion/trainees/post/sos-simplified-ophthalmic-statistics-part-3-which-statistical-test-should-i-use-if-any Accessed November 2021.

85. D.

Fig. 1.10 is a flowchart displaying common statistical tests and rules.

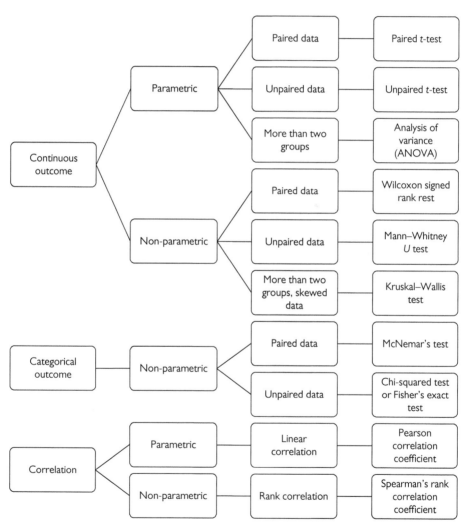

Figure 1.10 Flowchart for common statistical tests.

© Sohaib R. Rufai 2021.

Further reading

Bunce C, Young-Zvandasara T. Simplified Ophthalmic Statistics (SOS). Part 3: which statistical test should I use (if any)? *Eye News.* 2019;25(4):34–36. Available at: https://www.eyenews.uk.com/educat ion/trainees/post/sos-simplified-ophthalmic-statistics-part-3-which-statistical-test-should-i-use-if-any Accessed November 2021.

86. C.

Fig. 1.10 is a flowchart displaying common statistical tests and rules.

Further reading

Bunce C, Young-Zvandasara T. Simplified Ophthalmic Statistics (SOS). Part 3: which statistical test should I use (if any)? *Eye News.* 2019;25(4):34–36. Available at: https://www.eyenews.uk.com/educat ion/trainees/post/sos-simplified-ophthalmic-statistics-part-3-which-statistical-test-should-i-use-if-any Accessed November 2021.

87. B.

Recall bias can be caused by differences in the accuracy or completeness of recollections by participants regarding past events. Confirmation bias can be caused by the tendency to search for or favour information that confirms prior beliefs. Attrition bias can result due to unequal loss of participants from different arms of a trial. Selection bias can be caused by failure to achieve proper randomisation during participant selection.

Further reading

Denniston AKO, Moseley M, Murray PI. Chapter 26: Evidence-based ophthalmology. In: Denniston AKO, Murray PI. *Oxford Handbook of Ophthalmology.* Oxford University Press (2018).

88.

   I. B.

   II. D.

   III.C.

Equations for diagnostic accuracy testing:

$$Sensitivity = \frac{TP}{TP + FN}$$

$$Specificity = \frac{TN}{TN + FP}$$

$$PPV = \frac{TP}{TP + FP}$$

$$NPV = \frac{TN}{TN + FN}$$

$$Positive\ likelihood\ ratio = \frac{sensitivity}{1 - specificity}$$

$$Negative\ likelihood\ ratio = \frac{1 - sensitivity}{specificity}$$

$$Accuracy = \frac{TP + TN}{TP + TN + FP + FN}$$

Further reading

Denniston AKO, Moseley M, Murray PI. Chapter 26: Evidence-based ophthalmology. In: Denniston AKO, Murray PI. *Oxford Handbook of Ophthalmology*. Oxford University Press (2018).

Optics 2

1. **When excited by blue light, fluorescein sodium emits light of which wavelength range?**
    A. 450–460 nm
    B. 490–500 nm
    C. 520–530 nm
    D. 550–560 nm

2. **Regarding polarisation of light, which statement is MOST likely to be correct?**
    A. Polarising substances transmit light rays which are vibrating in multiple planes.
    B. A polarising medium increases radiant intensity but does not affect spectral composition.
    C. Birefringent substances split incident unpolarised light into two polarised beams travelling in different directions.
    D. Dichroic substances block transmission of light waves aligned with its structure by absorption.

3. **Regarding reflection, which statement is MOST likely to be correct?**
    A. If a plane mirror is rotated while light is incident upon the centre of rotation, the reflected ray is deviated through an angle equal to half the angle of rotation of the mirror.
    B. On reflection at a plane surface, the image of an object is erect, real, and laterally inverted.
    C. The anterior surface of the cornea acts as a convex mirror.
    D. The image formed by a concave mirror is virtual while that formed by a convex mirror is real.

4. **Which of the following refractive indices is INCORRECT?**
    A. Aqueous humour = 1.43
    B. Air = 1.00
    C. Crown glass = 1.52
    D. Cornea = 1.37

MCQs for FRCOphth Part 1. Sohaib R. Rufai, Oxford University Press. © Oxford University Press 2023.
DOI: 10.1093/oso/9780192843715.003.0002

5. **Regarding thin spherical lenses, where F$_1$ = first principal focus and F$_2$ = second principal focus, which statement is LEAST likely to be correct?**

    A. When the object is outside F$_1$, the image formed by a thin convex lens is virtual, inverted, and outside the second principal focus F$_2$.

    B. When the object is at F$_1$, the image formed by a thin convex lens is virtual, erect, and at infinity.

    C. When the object is inside F$_1$, the image formed by a thin convex lens is virtual, erect, magnified, and further from the lens than the object.

    D. When a real object is at any position, the image formed by a thin concave lens is virtual, erect, diminished, and inside F$_2$.

6. **Regarding the Maddox rod, which statement is LEAST likely to be true?**

    A. The Maddox rod can be used to diagnose extraocular muscle imbalance.

    B. The Maddox rod comprises weak convex cylindrical lenses mounted side by side in a trial lens.

    C. The glass of the Maddox rod is tinted red.

    D. To test for horizontal muscle imbalance, the Maddox rod must be placed horizontally.

7. **Regarding viewing a cross (+) through a lens, which statement is MOST likely to be correct?**

    A. When moving a concave lens side to side, the cross appears to move in the opposite direction.

    B. When moving a convex lens side to side, the cross appears to move in the same direction.

    C. When rotating a convex lens, 'scissoring' of the cross can be observed.

    D. A prism has no optical centre.

8. **Regarding the classification of astigmatism, which statement is MOST likely to be correct?**

    A. In simple myopic astigmatism, one line focus lies on the retina, while the other focus lies behind the retina.

    B. In mixed astigmatism, one line focus lies in front of the retina, while the other focus lies behind the retina.

    C. In simple hypermetropic astigmatism, rays in one meridian focus on the retina, while the other focus lies in front of the retina.

    D. In compound hypermetropic astigmatism, rays in all meridians come to a focus in front of the retina.

9. **Regarding the correction of aphakia with intraocular lenses (IOLs), which statement is MOST likely to be true?**

    A. The SRK formula is accurate for eyes with axial length shorter than 22 mm.

    B. Keratometry and B-scan ultrasonography are required to apply the SRK formula.

    C. The ideal postoperative refraction outcome for all patients should be emmetropia.

    D. Multifocal IOLs incorporate a near zone at or close to their centre.

10. **Regarding progressive addition lenses (PALs), which statement is MOST likely to be correct?**
    A. PALs with hard designs have a wider power progression corridor.
    B. PALs with soft designs tend to cause more pronounced aberrations close to the power progression corridor.
    C. PALs may be intolerable for prescriptions with a large cylinder.
    D. PALs represent a good solution for individuals requiring a wide near portion.

11. **Regarding the Galilean telescope, which statement is MOST likely to be true?**
    A. It consists of a concave objective lens and a convex eyepiece lens.
    B. The resulting image is inverted and magnified.
    C. It can be adapted to view near objects.
    D. It works by reducing the angle subtended by the object at the eye.

12. **Regarding retinoscopy, which statement is MOST likely to be true?**
    A. An image of the illuminated retina forms at the patient's nodal point.
    B. A patient with nystagmus should have their fellow eye completely occluded during retinoscopy.
    C. A diffuse bright red reflex is achieved when the movement of the reflex is infinitely fast.
    D. A working distance of 50 cm is equivalent to +1.5 dioptres.

13. **Regarding the Wollaston prism, which statement is LEAST likely to be true?**
    A. This prism consists of two quartz prisms cemented together.
    B. The two constituent prisms are positioned such that their optical axes are parallel.
    C. Quartz splits a single incident light beam into two polarised emerging beams.
    D. The two resulting images are sharp.

14. **Regarding the Goldmann applanation tonometer, which statement is LEAST likely to be true?**
    A. The applanation head houses two prisms with their bases in opposite directions.
    B. If the semicircles are viewed as widely overlapping, the applanation area is too small.
    C. The area of contact is elliptical in a patient with a high degree of corneal astigmatism.
    D. An abnormally thick central cornea may produce an artificially raised intraocular pressure reading.

15. **Regarding laser energy, which statement is LEAST likely to be true?**
    A. Laser light is coherent.
    B. Laser light is collimated.
    C. The process of pumping returns atoms in a laser active medium to the ground state.
    D. A laser producing 5 lumens of light may have a beam of luminous intensity equal to 500,000,000 candela.

16. **Regarding contact lenses, which statement is LEAST likely to be correct?**
    A. Contact lenses can reduce aniseikonia associated with anisometropia.
    B. Bandage contact lenses can be used for ocular surface disorders to relieve pain.
    C. Contact lenses move on blinking.
    D. Contact lenses can be used to perform electro-oculography.

Anatomy 2

17. **Which of the following represents the correct order of the bones of the medial orbital wall, from anterior to posterior?**
    A. Lacrimal bone, frontal process of maxilla, body of sphenoid, orbital plate of ethmoid
    B. Frontal process of maxilla, lacrimal bone, orbital plate of ethmoid, body of sphenoid
    C. Body of sphenoid, lacrimal bone, orbital plate of ethmoid, frontal process of maxilla
    D. Orbital plate of ethmoid, body of sphenoid, lacrimal bone, frontal process of maxilla

18. **Regarding the eyebrows, which statement is MOST likely to be true:**
    A. The medial end of the eyebrow lies above the medial end of the supraorbital margin, while the lateral end lies below the margin.
    B. Lowering the eyebrows is achieved by contracting the frontalis muscle.
    C. Raising the eyebrows is achieved by contracting the levator palpebrae.
    D. Drawing the eyebrows medially is achieved by contracting the corrugator supercilii.

19. **Regarding lacrimal drainage, which statement is MOST likely to be true?**
    A. The conjunctiva surrounding the punctum lacrimale is highly vascular.
    B. The lacrimal canaliculi are approximately 20 mm long.
    C. The lacrimal sac is approximately 12 mm long.
    D. The nasolacrimal duct is wider in its middle than at either end.

20. **From proximal to distal, which of the following options represents the correct order of rectus muscles in terms of distances between tendon insertions and the limbus?**
    A. Superior, medial, inferior, lateral
    B. Medial, inferior, lateral, superior
    C. Inferior, lateral, superior, medial
    D. Lateral, superior, medial, inferior

21. **What are the approximate horizontal and vertical dimensions of the cornea, respectively, in millimetres (mm)?**
    A. 11.7 mm, 10.6 mm
    B. 10.6 mm, 11.7 mm
    C. 7.7 mm, 6.9 mm
    D. 6.9 mm, 7.7 mm

22. **Which foramen of the skull transmits the middle meningeal artery?**
    A. Foramen lacerum
    B. Foramen spinosum
    C. Foramen rotundum
    D. Foramen ovale

23. **Regarding the choroid, which statement is LEAST likely to be true?**
    A. The choroid is thinnest at the posterior pole.
    B. The perichoroidal space is a potential space between the choroid and sclera.
    C. The choroid becomes continuous with the pia mater and arachnoid mater at the optic nerve.
    D. The outer surface of the choroid is roughened.

24. **Regarding the retina, which statement is MOST likely to be true?**
    A. It is approximately 0.1 mm thick near the optic disc.
    B. Its outer surface is in contact with the vitreous body.
    C. Its outer layer is derived from the inner layer of the optic cup.
    D. It extends more anteriorly on the medial side.

25. **Regarding ganglion cells, which statement is MOST likely to be true?**
    A. They are located in the outer retina.
    B. They are multipolar cells.
    C. They are first-order neurons in the visual pathway.
    D. Their diameter can vary from 50 to 70 micrometres.

26. **What is the approximate diameter of the adult human lens, in millimetres (mm)?**
    A. 8 mm
    B. 10 mm
    C. 12 mm
    D. 14 mm

27. Which of the following cranial nerves passes through the jugular foramen?

A. Facial nerve
B. Vestibulocochlear nerve
C. Vagus nerve
D. Hypoglossal nerve

28. Which of the following general visceral motor nuclei belongs to the facial nerve?

A. Dorsal motor nucleus
B. Edinger–Westphal nucleus
C. Lacrimal nucleus
D. Inferior salivatory nucleus

29. Regarding the optic disc, which statement is LEAST likely to be true?

A. It lies 3 mm nasally to the fovea.
B. It lies slightly above the posterior pole.
C. It is paler than the surrounding retina.
D. Its central part is flat.

30. By which day of embryological development does the lens vesicle separate from the surface ectoderm?

A. Day 29
B. Day 36
C. Day 39
D. Day 42

Physiology 2

Physiology of the eye and vision

31. Which of the following represents the correct order of tear film layers, from innermost to outermost?

A. Glycocalyx, lipid, mucous, aqueous
B. Glycocalyx, mucous, aqueous, lipid
C. Mucous, glycocalyx, aqueous, lipid
D. Mucous, glycocalyx, lipid, aqueous

32. **Regarding aqueous humour composition, which statement is LEAST likely to be true?**
   A. The protein concentration is lower in the central region of the anterior chamber than in the peripheral portion.
   B. The high ascorbate concentration of the aqueous may protect anterior ocular structures against oxidative damage induced by ultraviolet light.
   C. There is a higher glucose concentration in the aqueous relative to the plasma.
   D. There is a higher lactate concentration in the aqueous relative to the plasma.

33. **Which of the following does NOT represent a negative functional consequence of corneal ageing?**
   A. Decreased corneal sensation
   B. Decreased stromal strength
   C. Decreased tissue extensibility
   D. Impaired wound healing

34. **What is the primary structural protein found in the zonules of Zinn?**
   A. Collagen
   B. Laminin
   C. Entactin
   D. Fibrillin

35. **Regarding phototransduction, which of the following represents the correct photoisomerisation induced by light absorption?**
   A. All-trans retinal to 11-cis retinal
   B. 11-cis retinal to all-trans retinol
   C. All-trans retinal to 11-cis retinol
   D. 11-cis retinal to all-trans retinal

36. **The spacing between each of the bars of the 6/6 Snellen chart letter 'E' is equal to how many minutes of arc?**
   A. 1 minute
   B. 2 minutes
   C. 5 minutes
   D. 10 minutes

37. **Which of the following conditions is most likely to produce the highest magnitude of relative afferent pupillary defect (RAPD)?**
   A. Vitreous haemorrhage
   B. Central serous retinopathy
   C. Primary open-angle glaucoma
   D. Anterior ischaemic optic neuropathy

General physiology

38. Regarding osmosis, which statement is LEAST likely to be correct?

   A. Osmosis is the spontaneous net movement of solvent via a semipermeable membrane into a region of higher solute concentration.

   B. Osmotic pressure is amount of pressure that must be applied to a solution to prevent the inward flow of its pure solvent across a semipermeable membrane.

   C. One osmole is 1 gram molecular weight of osmotically active solute.

   D. Osmolarity is the osmolar concentration expressed as osmoles per kilogram of water.

39. Which of the following represents the first stage of the intrinsic pathway of the coagulation cascade?

   A. Action of activated factor X to form prothrombin activator

   B. Activation of factor XII and release of platelet phospholipids

   C. Activation of factor IX

   D. Activation of factor XI

40. Which of the following muscles are NOT involved in inspiration?

   A. External intercostals

   B. Anterior serrati

   C. Scaleni

   D. Abdominal recti

41. Regarding tactile receptors, which statement is MOST likely to be true?

   A. Merkel discs detect continuous contact of objects against the skin.

   B. Meissner's corpuscles are present in hairy areas of the skin.

   C. Ruffini endings detect tissue vibration.

   D. Pacinian corpuscles detect heavy prolonged touch and pressure.

42. Regarding filaments and junctions, which statement is MOST likely to be true?

   A. Zonulae occludentes form a barrier to paracellular diffusion of all molecules except water.

   B. Gap junctions occur at the blood–retinal barrier at the apex of the retinal pigment epithelium cell.

   C. Spot desmosomes are also known as zonulae adherentes.

   D. Claudin is a transmembrane protein with the ability to selectively permit the transport of charged ions.

43. Which of the following proteoglycans are NOT present in the sclera?

   A. Proteodermatan sulphate

   B. Proteokeratan sulphate

   C. Proteochondroitin sulphate

   D. Aggrecan

Pathology 2

General and ocular pathology

44. Which of the following pathological changes is NOT associated with diabetic retinopathy?

A. Increase in vascular endothelial growth factor and pigment epithelium-derived growth factor
B. Multilayering of the basement membrane of small vessels
C. Cataract
D. Vacuolation of the iris pigment epithelium

45. Regarding pyogenic infection, which statement is MOST likely to be correct?

A. Panophthalmitis may be complete by 24 hours.
B. Contaminated intraocular lenses are a common cause of acute exogenous endophthalmitis.
C. In metastatic endophthalmitis, neutrophils are the most predominant cell type.
D. Chronic corneal ulceration is a common cause of endophthalmitis.

46. Regarding herpes simplex keratitis, which statement is MOST likely to be true?

A. Type 1 herpes simplex virus can cause dendritic ulceration within the corneal endothelium.
B. Primary infection rarely occurs through the oral mucosa.
C. Complications of herpes simplex infection of the eye include disciform keratitis and secondary lipid keratopathy.
D. When reactivated, the virus can produce vesicle formation in the skin.

47. Regarding herpes zoster virus, which statement is LEAST likely to be true?

A. The virus can infect the ganglia and branches of the trigeminal nerve.
B. When reactivated, the virus can replicate and produce skin vesicles in the distribution of the affected nerve or branches thereof.
C. In herpes zoster ophthalmicus, the inflammatory process can involve the uveal tract, cornea, conjunctiva, and eyelids.
D. A monocytic infiltrate typically appears around the long and short ciliary nerves in herpes zoster ophthalmicus.

48. Regarding primary open-angle glaucoma, which statement is MOST likely to be true?

A. The optic cup enlarges more extensively in the horizontal plane than in the vertical plane as atrophy progresses.
B. Ischaemic optic atrophy is caused by occlusive disease in the anterior ciliary arteries.
C. The myocilin gene is located on chromosome 10.
D. The optineurin gene is involved in Golgi ribbon formation and exocytosis.

49. Regarding Stargardt's disease, which statement is MOST likely to be true?

A. In its early stages, lipofuscin and melanin accumulate in the retinal pigment epithelium.

B. In end-stage disease, the gliotic retina fuses with the retinal pigment epithelium.

C. On fundoscopy, the peripheral retina has a characteristic beaten-metal appearance.

D. Most cases result from mutations in the *SOD2* gene.

50. Regarding granular corneal dystrophy, which statement is MOST likely to be true?

A. It occasionally recurs in corneal grafts.

B. The endothelium is usually involved.

C. Birefringent hyaline bodies are found in the mid and anterior stroma and Bowman's layer.

D. It is inherited in an autosomal recessive manner.

51. Regarding malignant melanoma, which statement is MOST likely to be true?

A. Conjunctival melanomas carry worse prognosis in tumours thicker than 5 mm.

B. Iris melanomas are fast-growing nodular tumours.

C. Uveal melanomas are rarely unilateral.

D. Choroidal melanomas most commonly metastasise to the brain.

Microbiology

52. Regarding contact lens wear, which statement is LEAST likely to be true?

A. Long-term contact lens wear can suppress production of basal corneal epithelial cells by limbal stem cells.

B. Long-term contact lens wear can promote the proliferation and migration of corneal epithelial cells.

C. Extended wear soft contact lenses can trap microbes at the cell surface.

D. Extended wear soft contact lenses can reduce the flow and effectiveness of tears.

53. Which of the following represents the most common yeast responsible for corneal infections?

A. *Fusarium*

B. *Penicillium*

C. *Candida albicans*

D. *Aspergillus*

54. Regarding onchocerciasis, which statement is LEAST likely to be true?

A. The causative organism is *Onchocerca volvulus*—a filarial nematode.

B. Live microfilariae account for almost all associated immunopathology.

C. The host mounts a predominantly immunosuppressive response.

D. Blindness occurs due to ocular inflammation of the anterior and posterior segment.

Immunology

55. Regarding cells of the innate and acquired immune systems, which statement is LEAST likely to be true?

A. Mature T or B lymphocytes possess sparse cytoplasm and few mitochondria.

B. Natural killer cells possess abundant cytoplasm and abundant endoplasmic reticulum.

C. Macrophages possess few mitochondria and abundant lysosomes.

D. Monocytes possess abundant cytoplasm and few mitochondria.

56. Approximately what percentage of patients with acute anterior uveitis are human leukocyte antigen (HLA)-B27 positive?

A. 10%

B. 25%

C. 50%

D. 75%

Pharmacology and genetics 2

Pharmacology

57. Regarding pharmacokinetics, which statement is LEAST likely to be true?

A. The apparent volume of distribution is the volume of fluid required to contain the total amount of drug in the body at the same concentration present in the plasma.

B. The half-life of a drug is the time taken for the plasma drug concentration to halve following administration.

C. Estimation of drug clearance from the circulation is a less accurate way to assess the efficiency of drug clearance from the circulation as compared to drug half-life.

D. Bioavailability refers to the amount of oral drug dose that reaches systemic circulation and becomes available to the drug action site.

58. Which of the following scenarios is LEAST likely to prolong the residence time of ocular drugs in the fornix?

A. Nasolacrimal occlusion for 5 minutes after topically applying the drug.

B. Using ointment rather than solution as a vehicle.

C. Surgically correcting ectropion.

D. Formulation at alkaline pH.

59. Which of the following is LEAST likely to be a systemic side effect of topical anti-muscarinic drugs?

A. Sweating

B. Facial flushing

C. Dry mouth

D. Bradycardia

60. **Regarding ocular toxicity from systemic administration of drugs, which statement is LEAST likely to be true?**
    A. Chloroquine has a high affinity for binding to melanin.
    B. Amiodarone is not a photosensitising agent.
    C. Long-term steroid use can cause cataracts.
    D. Chloroquine retinopathy is usually seen in patients receiving the drug for more than 1 year.

61. **Which of the following represents the major neurotransmitter of the parasympathetic nervous system?**
    A. Acetylcholine
    B. Noradrenaline
    C. Adrenaline
    D. Norepinephrine

62. **Which of the following histamine receptor antagonists acts on H$_1$-receptors?**
    A. Ranitidine
    B. Ciproxifan
    C. Cetirizine
    D. Thioperamide

Genetics

63. **Which is the first stage of the prophase of the first meiotic division?**
    A. Diplotene
    B. Pachytene
    C. Zygotene
    D. Leptotene

64. **Regarding numerical chromosomal abnormalities, which statement is LEAST likely to be true?**
    A. Aneuploidy can result from delayed movement during metaphase.
    B. In triploidy, there are 69 chromosomes in total.
    C. Turner syndrome can result from meiotic aneuploidy.
    D. Robertsonian translocation can cause Down syndrome.

65. **Which human leukocyte antigen (HLA) allele is strongly associated with birdshot chorioretinopathy?**
    A. HLA-B27
    B. HLA-DR4
    C. HLA-B51
    D. HLA-A29

66. **Which of the following gene mutations is associated with idiopathic infantile nystagmus?**
    A. *OCA2*
    B. *CNGA3*
    C. *PAX6*
    D. *FRMD7*

67. **Regarding gene therapy strategies, which statement is LEAST likely to be true?**
    A. Gene augmentation therapy aims to restore normal phenotype by supplying more copies of the normal gene.
    B. Targeting mutation correction can be achieved using ribozymes, which block gene transcription.
    C. Targeted inhibition of gene expression can be used in diseases that demonstrate excessive expression of gene product.
    D. In targeted killing of specific cells, protein kills cells by interfering with cell cycling and survival.

68. **Regarding the ubiquitin-proteosome pathway, which statement is LEAST likely to be true?**
    A. This pathway maintains cellular homeostasis.
    B. Proteosomes degrade proteins, which become covalently bonded to ubiquitin.
    C. Ubiquitin plays a role in protecting phosphorylated cyclins and cyclin inhibitors.
    D. Lactacystin is a proteasome inhibitor.

Investigations 2

69. **Regarding Maddox tests for symptomatic phorias, which statement is MOST likely to be true?**
    A. The Maddox wing test is used for torsional phorias.
    B. Two red Maddox rods are used in the double Maddox rod test.
    C. Distance correction is not required for the Maddox rod test.
    D. The Maddox rod is positioned vertically for vertical phorias.

70. **Regarding the prism cover test, how should the prism be orientated for an exotropia?**
    A. Base-up
    B. Base-down
    C. Base-in
    D. Base-out

71. **Regarding the Hirschberg test, what is indicated by a temporal corneal reflection?**
    A. Hypertropia
    B. Hypotropia
    C. Exotropia
    D. Esotropia

72. **Which of the following conditions is LEAST likely to cause constriction of the peripheral visual fields?**
    A. Central retinal artery occlusion
    B. Optic nerve coloboma
    C. Retinitis pigmentosa
    D. Bilateral panretinal photocoagulation

73. **Regarding corneal topography, which statement is LEAST likely to be true?**
    A. When using relative scales, curvature maps compare the data against set ranges.
    B. The average cornea in adults has with-the-rule astigmatism.
    C. Corneal topography can detect pellucid marginal degeneration.
    D. Scheimpflug imaging enables evaluation of the posterior corneal surface.

74. **Which of the following is LEAST likely to represent a side effect of fundus fluorescein angiography?**
    A. Nausea and vomiting
    B. Transient discolouration of skin
    C. Pruritus
    D. Staining of stool

75. **In indocyanine green (ICG) angiography, how long is the late mid-phase?**
    A. 15–30 minutes
    B. 3–15 minutes
    C. 1–3 minutes
    D. 2–60 seconds

76. **What is the layer marked with an arrow on this optical coherence tomography (OCT) image?**

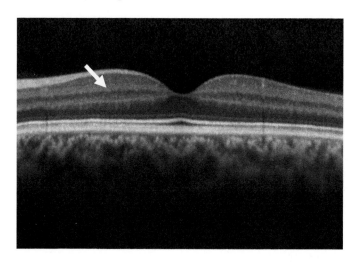

A. Outer plexiform layer
B. Inner nuclear layer
C. Ganglion cell layer
D. Inner plexiform layer

77. **Regarding the full-field electroretinogram (ffERG), which of the following conditions is MOST likely to produce a normal a-wave and reduced scotopic b-wave?**

A. Total retinal detachment
B. Rod-cone dystrophy
C. Congenital stationary night blindness
D. Achromatopsia

78. **Regarding the multifocal electroretinogram (mfERG), which statement is LEAST likely to be true?**

A. It produces a topographical functional map of the retina.
B. Areas of the retina are stimulated with unchanging stimuli.
C. It can be converted to a three-dimensional map of retinal function that represents the hill of vision.
D. It is helpful when retinal dysfunction is localised or patchy.

79. **Regarding the pattern electroretinogram (ERG), in a normal subject, when would the negative deflection be expected?**

A. 135 milliseconds
B. 95 milliseconds
C. 75 milliseconds
D. 50 milliseconds

Miscellaneous 2

80. **In hypothesis testing, what does the p-value represent?**
    A. Significance level
    B. Power
    C. Probability of obtaining the observed data or data that were more extreme due to chance if the null hypothesis were true
    D. Effect size

81. **For which study type should the STROBE reporting guideline be used?**
    A. Systematic review
    B. Randomised controlled trial
    C. Diagnostic accuracy study
    D. Cohort study

82. **What is the mean value of the following numbers?**
    32, 44, 44, 74, 76
    A. 44
    B. 54
    C. 64
    D. 74

83. **In a normally distributed dataset, approximately what percentage of values lie within one standard deviation of the mean?**
    A. 50%
    B. 60%
    C. 65%
    D. 68%

84. **Which of the following is NOT a leading cause of blindness globally, according to the World Health Organization?**
    A. Trachoma
    B. Diabetic retinopathy
    C. Corneal opacity
    D. Retinitis pigmentosa

85. **What is the MOST appropriate statistical test to use for two groups where the outcome measure is continuous and the data are parametric and paired?**
    A. Analysis of variance
    B. Paired t-test
    C. McNemar's test
    D. Chi-squared test

86. **Which of the following is a non-parametric measure of rank correlation between two variables?**
    A. Pearson correlation coefficient
    B. Pearson's r
    C. Pearson product-moment correlation coefficient
    D. Spearman's rank correlation coefficient

87. **Which of the following options represents the MOST likely cause of lead-time bias?**
    A. Earlier diagnosis of a disease falsely makes it seem like affected patients are surviving longer.
    B. The tendency to favour recent events over older events.
    C. Systematic differences between groups in how outcomes are determined.
    D. The outcome of the study influences the decision whether or not to publish it.

88. **Regarding diagnostic accuracy testing, where T = true, F = false, P = positives, and N = negatives:**

    I. Which of the following equations is used to calculate specificity?

    A. $\dfrac{TP}{TP+FN}$

    B. $\dfrac{TP}{TP+FP}$

    C. $\dfrac{TN}{TN+FN}$

    D. $\dfrac{TN}{TN+FP}$

    II. Which of the following equations is used to calculate sensitivity?

    A. $\dfrac{TN}{TN+FN}$

    B. $\dfrac{TN}{TN+FP}$

    C. $\dfrac{TP}{TP+FN}$

    D. $\dfrac{TP}{TP+FP}$

    III. Which of the following equations is used to calculate positive predictive value (PPV)?

    A. $\dfrac{TN}{TN+FP}$

    B. $\dfrac{TN}{TN+FN}$

    C. $\dfrac{TP}{TP+FP}$

    D. $\dfrac{TP}{TP+FN}$

Optics 2

1. C.

Fluorescein sodium emits yellow-green light (520–530 nm) when excited by blue light (465–490 nm).

Further reading

Chapter 1: Properties of light and visual function. In: Elkington AR, Frank HJ, Greaney MJ. *Clinical Optics*. Blackwell Science (1999).

2. C.

Polarising substances only transmit light rays which are vibrating in **one** plane. A polarising medium **reduces** radiant intensity but does not affect spectral composition. Dichroic substances block transmission of light waves **not** aligned with its structure by absorption.

Further reading

Chapter 1: Properties of light and visual function. In: Elkington AR, Frank HJ, Greaney MJ. *Clinical Optics*. Blackwell Science (1999).

3. C.

If a plane mirror is rotated while light is incident upon the centre of rotation, the reflected ray is deviated through an angle equal to twice the angle of rotation of the mirror. On reflection at a plane surface, the image of an object is erect, virtual, and laterally inverted. The image formed by a concave mirror is real while that formed by a convex mirror is virtual.

Further reading

Chapter 2: Reflection of light. In: Elkington AR, Frank HJ, Greaney MJ. *Clinical Optics*. Blackwell Science (1999).

4. A.

The refractive index of aqueous humour is approximately 1.33. See Table 1.2 (p. xxx) for refractive indices of the eye.

Further reading

Chapter 3: Refraction of light. In: Elkington AR, Frank HJ, Greaney MJ. *Clinical Optics*. Blackwell Science (1999).

5. A.

When the object is outside F_1, the image formed by a thin convex lens is REAL, inverted, and outside the second principal focus F_2. Other options are true. Fig. 2.1 displays three ray diagrams for images formed by thin convex lenses, depending on the position of the object. Fig. 2.2 displays a ray diagram for the image formed by a thin concave lens.

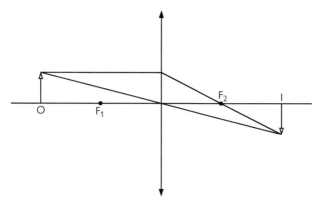

(a) O outside F1; I = real, inverted, and outside F_2 (RIO).

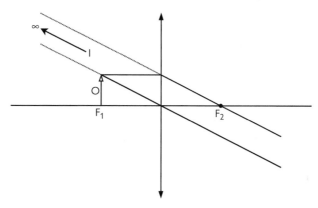

(b) O at F1; I = virtual, erect, and at infinity (VE∞).

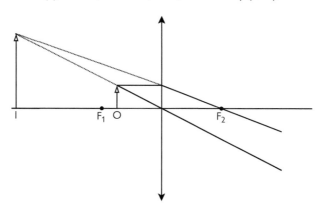

(c) O inside F1; I = virtual, erect, magnified (VEM), and further from lens than O.

Figure 2.1 Image formation by thin convex lens, where object is outside first principal focus (a), at first principal focus (b), and inside first principal focus (c). Key: O = object; I = image; F_1 = first principal focus; F_2 = second principal focus.

Figure courtesy of Mr Umar Ahmed, Medical Student, Imperial College London.

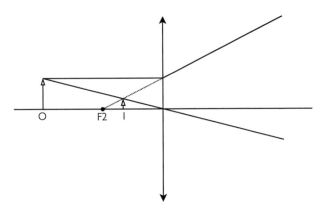

Figure 2.2 Image formation by thin concave lens, where object is at any position. The image is virtual, erect, diminished (VED) and inside the second principal focus. Key: O = object; I = image; F_1 = first principal focus; F_2 = second principal focus.

Figure courtesy of Mr Umar Ahmed, Medical Student, Imperial College London.

Further reading

Chapter 5: Spherical lenses. In: Elkington AR, Frank HJ, Greaney MJ. *Clinical Optics*. Blackwell Science (1999).

6. B.

The Maddox comprises a series of powerful convex cylindrical lenses mounted side by side in a trial lens.

Further reading

Chapter 6: Astigmatic lenses. In: Elkington AR, Frank HJ, Greaney MJ. *Clinical Optics*. Blackwell Science (1999).

7. D.

A concave lens creates a 'with movement' whereas a convex lens creates an 'against movement', with respect to the cross. When rotating an astigmatic lens, scissoring of the cross can be observed.

Further reading

Chapter 7: Optical prescriptions, spectacle lenses. In: Elkington AR, Frank HJ, Greaney MJ. *Clinical Optics*. Blackwell Science (1999).

8. B.

In simple myopic astigmatism, one line focus lies on the retina, while the other focus lies in front of the retina. In simple hypermetropic astigmatism, rays in one meridian focus on the retina, while the other focus lies behind the retina. In compound hypermetropic astigmatism, rays in all meridians come to a focus behind the retina.

Further reading

Chapter 10: Optics of ametropia. In: Elkington AR, Frank HJ, Greaney MJ. *Clinical Optics*. Blackwell Science (1999).

9. D.

The original SRK formula is inaccurate for eyes of axial length under 22 mm or over 24.5 mm. A recent systematic review by Wang and colleagues (2018) concluded that the Haigis formula is superior in predicting IOL power in short eyes. Keratometry and A-scan ultrasonography are required to measure corneal curvature (i.e. refractive power) and axial length, both required by the SRK formula. The ideal postoperative refraction outcome for all patients is not always emmetropia, e.g. lifelong myopes and/or those who conduct close working (e.g. watchmakers) often prefer to be left slightly myopic after cataract surgery, while others may prefer monovision (one eye for distance and the other for near). Multifocal IOLs incorporate a near zone at or close to their centre, due to pupil constriction for near vision.

Further reading

Chapter 10: Optics of ametropia. In: Elkington AR, Frank HJ, Greaney MJ. *Clinical Optics*. Blackwell Science (1999).

Wang Q, Jiang W, Lin T, et al. Meta-analysis of accuracy of intraocular lens power calculation formulas in short eyes. *Clinical & Experimental Ophthalmology*. 2018 May;46(4):356–363.

10. C.

PALs with hard designs have wider distance and near portions and a narrower power progression corridor, near which aberrations can occur. On the other hand, newer soft designs have a wider power progression corridor and smaller distance and nearer portions—these tend to be better tolerated. Individuals requiring a wider near portion are unlikely to be satisfied by PALs.

Further reading

Chapter 11: Presbyopia. In: Elkington AR, Frank HJ, Greaney MJ. *Clinical Optics*. Blackwell Science (1999).

11. C.

The Galilean telescope consists of a convex objective lens and concave eyepiece lens. The resulting image is erect and magnified. It can be adapted to view near or distant objects. It works by increasing the angle subtended by the object at the eye. Fig. 2.3 is a ray diagram demonstrating the optics of the Galilean telescope.

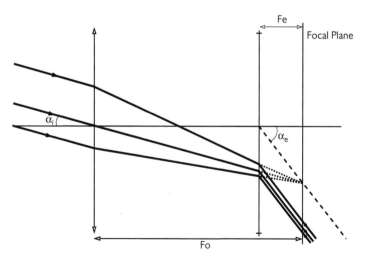

Figure 2.3 The Galilean telescope. Key: α_i = angle of incidence; α_e = angle of emergence; Fe = focal length of eyepiece lens; Fo = focal length of objective lens.

Figure courtesy of Mr Umar Ahmed, Medical Student, Imperial College London.

Further reading

Chapter 13: Optics of low vision aids. In: Elkington AR, Frank HJ, Greaney MJ. *Clinical Optics.* Blackwell Science (1999).

12. C.

An image of the illuminated retina forms at the patient's far point. A patient with nystagmus should have their fellow eye fogged with a high plus lens during retinoscopy, as complete occlusion may make their nystagmus worse and reduce visual acuity in the tested eye. A working distance of 50 cm is equivalent to +2 dioptres, whereas a working distance of 66 cm (2/3 m) is approximately equivalent to +1.50 dioptres. The refractionist's working distance must be subtracted from the prescription.

Further reading

Chapter 14: Instruments. In: Elkington AR, Frank HJ, Greaney MJ. *Clinical Optics.* Blackwell Science (1999).

Chapter 16: Practical clinical refraction. In: Elkington AR, Frank HJ, Greaney MJ. *Clinical Optics.* Blackwell Science (1999).

13. B.

The two constituent prisms are positioned such that their optical axes are perpendicular. Fig. 2.4 shows four ray diagrams displaying the optical properties of the following prisms: Wollaston, Porro, Dove, and right angle.

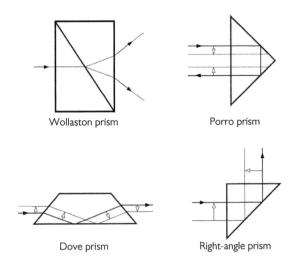

Wollaston prism   Porro prism

Dove prism   Right-angle prism

Figure 2.4 Wollaston, Porro, Dove, and right-angle prisms.

Figure courtesy of Mr Umar Ahmed, Medical Student, Imperial College London.

Further reading

Chapter 14: Instruments. In: Elkington AR, Frank HJ, Greaney MJ. *Clinical Optics.* Blackwell Science (1999).

14. B.

If the semicircles are far apart, the applanation area is too small. If the semicircle areas only just overlap one another, the applanation area is correct (3.06 mm in diameter). If the semicircles widely overlap one another, the applanation area is too large. Fig. 2.5 is a schematic displaying the appearance of the semicircles viewed using the Goldmann applanation tonometer when the area is too small, correct, and too large.

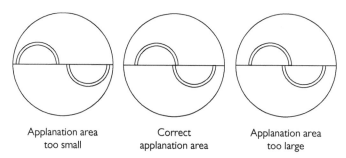

| Applanation area
too small | Correct
applanation area | Applanation area
too large |

Figure 2.5 Semicircles viewed when performing Goldmann applanation tonometry.

Figure courtesy of Dr Sohaib Rufai. © Sohaib R. Rufai 2021.

Further reading

Chapter 14: Instruments. In: Elkington AR, Frank HJ, Greaney MJ. *Clinical Optics.* Blackwell Science (1999).

15. C.

The process of pumping delivers energy to atoms in a laser active medium. The atoms absorb this energy, which elevates their electrons from their ground state (most stable) to a higher energy level.

Further reading

Chapter 15: Lasers. In: Elkington AR, Frank HJ, Greaney MJ. *Clinical Optics.* Blackwell Science (1999).

16. D.

Contact lenses can indeed reduce or eliminate aniseikonia (difference in perceived size of images) caused by anisometropia and high degrees of astigmatism. Bandage contact lenses can be used for ocular surface disorders to protect the ocular surface, promote healing, and relieve pain. Contact lenses move slightly on blinking, but a correctly fitted contact lens should not move excessively. A special contact lens with a built-in electrode is used to perform electroretinography, not electro-oculography.

Further reading

Chapter 12: Contact lenses. In: Elkington AR, Frank HJ, Greaney MJ. *Clinical Optics.* Blackwell Science (1999).

Anatomy 2

17. B.

From anterior to posterior, the medial orbital wall comprises the frontal process of **M**axilla, **L**acrimal bone, orbital plate of **E**thmoid, and body of **S**phenoid. A useful mnemonic to remember this order is: 'My Little Eye Sits in the orbit'. The orbital plate of the ethmoid forms the largest part of the medial orbital wall.

Further reading

Chapter 1: Anatomy of the eye and orbit. In: Forrester JV, Dick AD, McMenamin PG, Roberts F, Pearlman E. *The Eye: Basic Sciences in Practice* (4th Edition). Elsevier (2016).

Chapter 3: The orbital cavity. In: Snell RS, Lemp MA. *Clinical Anatomy of the Eye* (2nd Edition). John Wiley and Sons (1998).

18. D.

The lateral end of the eyebrow lies above the supraorbital margin, while the medial end lies below the margin. Lowering the eyebrows is achieved by contracting the orbital portion of the orbicularis oculi, while raising the eyebrows is achieved by contracting the frontalis muscle. The corrugator supercilii draws the eyebrows medially when contracted, hence it is the 'frowning' muscle.

Further reading

Chapter 5: The ocular appendages. In: Snell RS, Lemp MA. *Clinical Anatomy of the Eye* (2nd Edition). John Wiley and Sons (1998).

19. C.

The conjunctiva surrounding the punctum lacrimale is somewhat avascular, hence it appears pale red. The lacrimal canaliculi are approximately 10 mm long. The nasolacrimal duct is approximately 18 mm long and is narrower in the middle as compared to either end.

Further reading

Chapter 5: The ocular appendages. In: Snell RS, Lemp MA. *Clinical Anatomy of the Eye* (2nd Edition). John Wiley and Sons (1998).

20. B.

From proximal to distal, the correct order of rectus muscles in terms of distances between tendon insertions and the limbus is as follows: **M**edial (5.5 mm), **I**nferior (6.5 mm), **L**ateral (6.9 mm), and **S**uperior (7.7 mm). You can remember these with the acronym **MILS**. These insertions form an imaginary spiral called the spiral of Tillaux. Fig. 2.6 is a schematic displaying the spiral of Tillaux. Please note that different textbooks quote slightly different measurements.

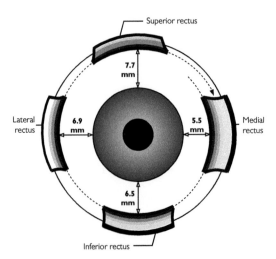

Figure 2.6 The spiral of Tillaux.

Figure courtesy of Mr Umar Ahmed, Medical Student, Imperial College London.

Further reading

Chapter 6: The eyeball. In: Snell RS, Lemp MA. *Clinical Anatomy of the Eye* (2nd Edition). John Wiley and Sons (1998).

21. A.

The cornea approximately measures 11.7 mm horizontally and 10.6 mm vertically, while its radius of curvature is 7.7 mm for the anterior surface and 6.9 mm for the posterior surface.

Further reading

Chapter 6: The eyeball. In: Snell RS, Lemp MA. *Clinical Anatomy of the Eye* (2nd Edition). John Wiley and Sons (1998).

22. B.

The foramen spinosum perforates the greater wing of sphenoid, posterolateral to the foramen ovale. It transmits the middle meningeal artery and vein, plus the meningeal branch of the mandibular nerve.

Further reading

Chapter 1: An overview of the anatomy of the skull. In: Snell RS, Lemp MA. *Clinical Anatomy of the Eye* (2nd Edition). John Wiley and Sons (1998).

Chapter 1: Anatomy of the eye and orbit. In: Forrester JV, Dick AD, McMenamin PG, Roberts F, Pearlman E. *The Eye: Basic Sciences in Practice* (4th Edition). Elsevier (2016).

23. A.

The choroid is thickest at the posterior pole and thinnest proximal to the optic disc.

Further reading

Chapter 6: The eyeball. In: Snell RS, Lemp MA. *Clinical Anatomy of the Eye* (2nd Edition). John Wiley and Sons (1998).

24. D.

The retina is approximately 0.1 mm thick at the ora serrata and 0.56 mm thick near the optic disc. Its inner surface is in contact with the vitreous body whereas its outer surface is in contact with Bruch's membrane. Its inner layer is derived from the inner layer of the optic cup, while its outer layer is derived from the outer layer of the optic cup.

Further reading

Chapter 6: The eyeball. In: Snell RS, Lemp MA. *Clinical Anatomy of the Eye* (2nd Edition). John Wiley and Sons (1998).

25. B.

Ganglion cells are located in the inner retina. They are second-order neurons in the visual pathway. Their diameter can vary from 10 to 30 micrometres.

Further reading

Chapter 6: The eyeball. In: Snell RS, Lemp MA. *Clinical Anatomy of the Eye* (2nd Edition). John Wiley and Sons (1998).

26. B.

The human lens measures approximately 6.5 mm at birth and grows to approximately 10 mm in adults.

Further reading

Chapter 6: The eyeball. In: Snell RS, Lemp MA. *Clinical Anatomy of the Eye* (2nd Edition). John Wiley and Sons (1998).

27. C.

The jugular foramen transmits the following cranial nerves: glossopharyngeal, vagus, and accessory. Table 2.1 summarises the functional components and foramina of the cranial nerves.

Table 2.1 Cranial nerves: functional components and foramina

Cranial nerve	Components	Foramen
Olfactory (I)	Sensory: SVA	Cribriform plate
Optic (II)	Sensory: SSA	Optic canal
Oculomotor (III)	Motor: GSE, GVE	Superior orbital fissure
Trochlear (IV)	Motor: GSE	Superior orbital fissure
Trigeminal (V) **Ophthalmic division (V₁)** **Maxillary division (V₂)** **Mandibular division (V₃)**	Sensory: GSA Sensory: GSA Motor: SVE	Superior orbital fissure Foramen rotundum Foramen ovale
Abducens (VI)	Motor: GSE	Superior orbital fissure
Facial (VII)	Motor: SVE Sensory: SVA Secretomotor: GVE	Internal acoustic meatus, facial canal, stylomastoid canal
Vestibulocochlear (VIII)	Sensory: SSA	Internal acoustic meatus
Glossopharyngeal (IX)	Motor: SVE Secretomotor: GVE Sensory: GVA, SVA, GSA	Jugular foramen
Vagus (X)	Motor: GVE, SVE Sensory: GVA, SVA, GSA	Jugular foramen
Accessory (XI)	Motor: SVE	Jugular foramen
Hypoglossal (XII)	Motor: GSE	Hypoglossal canal

Key: GSA = general somatic afferent; GSE = general somatic efferent; GVA = general visceral afferent; GVE = general visceral efferent; SSA = special somatic afferent; SVA = special visceral afferent; SVE = special visceral efferent.

Further reading

Chapter 10: Cranial nerves—part 1: the nerves directly associated with the eye and orbit. In: Snell RS, Lemp MA. *Clinical Anatomy of the Eye* (2nd Edition). John Wiley and Sons (1998).

28. C.

The general visceral motor nuclei providing the cranial outflow of the parasympathetic nervous system are as follows: Edinger–Westphal nucleus: oculomotor nerve; superior salivatory and lacrimal nuclei: facial nerve; inferior salivatory nucleus: glossopharyngeal nerve; dorsal motor nucleus: vagus nerve.

Further reading

Chapter 10: Cranial nerves—part 1: the nerves directly associated with the eye and orbit. In: Snell RS, Lemp MA. *Clinical Anatomy of the Eye* (2nd Edition). John Wiley and Sons (1998).

29. D.

The edges of the optic disc are flat or slightly raised, whereas its central part has a slight depression in which the central retinal vessels enter/exit the eye.

Further reading

Chapter 13: The visual pathway. In: Snell RS, Lemp MA. *Clinical Anatomy of the Eye* (2nd Edition). John Wiley and Sons (1998).

30. B.

By day 36 of embryological development, the lens vesicle separates from the surface ectoderm.

Further reading

Chapter 1: Anatomy of the eye and orbit. In: Forrester JV, Dick AD, McMenamin PG, Roberts F, Pearlman E. *The Eye: Basic Sciences in Practice* (4th Edition). Elsevier (2016).

Physiology 2

Physiology of the eye and vision

31. B.

The correct order of tear film layers, from innermost to outermost, is as follows: glycocalyx, mucous, aqueous, lipid.

Further reading

Dartt DA. Chapter 15: Formation and function of the tear film. In: Levin LA, Nilsson SFE, Ver Hoeve J, et al. *Adler's Physiology of the Eye* (11th Edition). Elsevier (2011).

32. C.

There are slightly lower concentrations of glucose, urea, and non-protein nitrogen in the aqueous relative to the plasma. The concentration of protein is 20 times less in the aqueous relative to the plasma. There are higher concentrations of ascorbate, lactate, and chloride, plus certain amino acids, in the aqueous relative to the plasma.

Further reading

Gabelt BT and Kaufman PL. Chapter 11: Production and flow of aqueous humor. In: Levin LA, Nilsson SFE, Ver Hoeve J, et al. *Adler's Physiology of the Eye* (11th Edition). Elsevier (2011).

33. B.

Strength, stiffness, and toughness of the corneal stroma increases with age, due to enzymatic maturation and glycation-induced cross-linking of collagen fibrils. Thus, keratoconus is rarely seen in individuals above 40 years of age.

Further reading

Dawson DG, Ubels JL, Edelhauser HF. Chapter 4: Cornea and sclera. In: Levin LA, Nilsson SFE, Ver Hoeve J, et al. *Adler's Physiology of the Eye* (11th Edition). Elsevier (2011).

34. D.

Fibrillin is the primary structural protein found in the zonules of Zinn (also termed the suspensory ligaments). Hence, patients with Marfan syndrome often have lens dislocation, due to mutations in the fibrillin gene.

Further reading

Beebe DC. Chapter 5: The lens. In: Levin LA, Nilsson SFE, Ver Hoeve J, et al. *Adler's Physiology of the Eye* (11th Edition). Elsevier (2011).

35. D.

The bound 11-cis retinal chromophore enters its excited stated following light absorption, undergoing photoisomerisation from **11-cis retinal** to **all-trans retinal**.

Further reading

Gross AK, Wensel TG. Chapter 18: Biochemical cascade of phototransduction. In: Levin LA, Nilsson SFE, Ver Hoeve J, et al. *Adler's Physiology of the Eye* (11th Edition). Elsevier (2011).

36. A.

To correctly identify the letters of the Snellen chart, one must be able to see the clear spacing between the black elements of the letters. Fig. 2.7 displays the correct design of the 6/6 'E' Snellen chart letter, in minutes of arc.

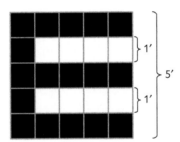

Figure 2.7 A 6/6 'E' Snellen chart letter. The spacing between each of the bars of the 'E' is equal to 1 minute of arc (1'), while the entire height of the 'E' is equal to 5 minutes of arc (5').

Figure courtesy of Dr Sohaib Rufai. © Sohaib R Rufai 2021.

Further reading

Chapter 5: Physiology of vision and the visual system. In: Forrester JV, Dick AD, McMenamin PG, Roberts F, Pearlman E. *The Eye: Basic Sciences in Practice* (4th Edition). Elsevier (2016).

37. D.

Dense vitreous haemorrhage can produce 0.6–1.2 log units RAPD, depending on the density of the haemorrhage. Central serous retinopathy can produce 0.3 log units RAPD, depending on the area of retina involved. Primary open-angle glaucoma usually does not produce RAPD, provided the damage to both eyes is symmetrical; the degree of visual field asymmetry between the eyes is correlated with the log unit RAPD. Anterior ischaemic optic neuropathy can produce 0.6–2.7 log units RAPD, depending on the extent and location of the visual field defect.

Further reading

Kardon R. Chapter 25: Regulation of light through the pupil. In: Levin LA, Nilsson SFE, Ver Hoeve J, et al. *Adler's Physiology of the Eye* (11th Edition). Elsevier (2011).

General physiology

38. D.

Osmolarity is the osmolar concentration expressed as osmoles per litre of solution (not per kilogram of water).

Further reading

Chapter 2: The cell and its functions. In: Hall JE. *Guyton and Hall Textbook of Medical Physiology* (13th Edition). Elsevier (2016).

39. B.

The intrinsic pathway of the coagulation cascade can be summarised as follows:

1. Blood trauma causes activation of factor XII and release of platelet phospholipids.
2. Activation of factor XI by activated factor XII.
3. Activation of factor IX by activated factor XI.
4. Activation of factor X by activated factor XI, activated factor VIII, platelet phospholipids, and factor III from traumatised platelets.
5. Action of activated factor X to form prothrombin activator.

Further reading

Chapter 37: Haemostasis and blood coagulation. In: Hall JE. *Guyton and Hall Textbook of Medical Physiology* (13th Edition). Elsevier (2016).

40. D.

Muscles of inspiration elevate the rib cage while muscles of expiration depress the rib cage. The external intercostals elevate the rib cage. The sternocleidomastoid muscles lift the sternum upwards. The anterior serrati lifts many of the ribs while the scaleni lift the first two ribs. The abdominal recti pull the lower ribs downwards and compress the abdominal contents upwards to raise the diaphragm, while the internal intercostals pull the rib cage downwards.

Further reading

Chapter 38: Pulmonary ventilation. In: Hall JE. *Guyton and Hall Textbook of Medical Physiology* (13th Edition). Elsevier (2016).

41. A.

Merkel discs detect continuous contact of objects against the skin. Meissner's corpuscles are present in non-hairy areas of the skin. Ruffini endings detect heavy prolonged touch and stretch. Pacinian corpuscles detect tissue vibration.

Further reading

Chapter 48: Somatic sensations: I. General organization, the tactile and positional senses. In: Hall JE. *Guyton and Hall Textbook of Medical Physiology* (13th Edition). Elsevier (2016).

42. D.

Zonulae occludens (also known as tight junctions) form a barrier to paracellular diffusion of all molecules, **including** water and ions. Zonulae occludens occur at the blood–retinal barrier at the apex of the retinal pigment epithelium cell and at the blood–aqueous barrier of the ciliary body. There are two types of desmosomes: spot desmosomes (single site), also known as macula adherens, and belt desmosomes (ring round the apex of the cell), also known as zonulae adherens.

Further reading

Chapter 4: Biochemistry and cell biology. In: Forrester JV, Dick AD, McMenamin PG, Roberts F, Pearlman E. *The Eye: Basic Sciences in Practice* (5th Edition). Elsevier (2021).

43. B.

Proteodermatan sulphate and proteochondroitin sulphate (of the SLR type) represent the major proteoglycans of the sclera. Others include aggrecan, decorin, biglycan, and proline–arginine–rich and leucine-rich repeat (PRELP). There are no proteokeratan sulphates in the sclera.

Further reading

Chapter 4: Biochemistry and cell biology. In: Forrester JV, Dick AD, McMenamin PG, Roberts F, Pearlman E. *The Eye: Basic Sciences in Practice* (5th Edition). Elsevier (2021).

Pathology 2

General and ocular pathology

44. A

In diabetic retinopathy, retinal hypoxia alters the balance of important growth factors. Vascular endothelial growth factor (VEGF) and placental growth factor (PIGF) are both increased. Pigment epithelium-derived growth factor (PEDF) is decreased. VEGF and PIGF are angiogenic whereas PEDF is anti-angiogenic.

Further reading

Chapter 9: Pathology. In: Forrester JV, Dick AD, McMenamin PG, Roberts F, Pearlman E. *The Eye: Basic Sciences in Practice* (4th Edition). Elsevier (2016).

45. C

Panophthalmitis may be complete by 48 hours. Contaminated intraocular lenses, commonly used in cataract surgery, are a common cause of late, low-grade bacterial endophthalmitis. Chronic corneal ulceration, debility, and immunosuppression are rare causes of endophthalmitis.

Further reading

Chapter 9: Pathology. In: Forrester JV, Dick AD, McMenamin PG, Roberts F, Pearlman E. *The Eye: Basic Sciences in Practice* (4th Edition). Elsevier (2016).

46. C.

Type 1 herpes simplex virus can cause dendritic ulceration within the corneal epithelium. Primary infection often occurs through the oral mucosa, as well as the lips and facial skin. When reactivated, the virus travels along the sensory nerves to the corneal epithelium. Option D is applicable to herpes zoster ophthalmicus.

Further reading

Chapter 9: Pathology. In: Forrester JV, Dick AD, McMenamin PG, Roberts F, Pearlman E. *The Eye: Basic Sciences in Practice* (4th Edition). Elsevier (2016).

47. D.

A lymphocytic infiltrate typically appears around the long and short ciliary nerves in herpes zoster ophthalmicus.

Further reading

Chapter 9: Pathology. In: Forrester JV, Dick AD, McMenamin PG, Roberts F, Pearlman E. *The Eye: Basic Sciences in Practice* (4th Edition). Elsevier (2016).

48. D.

The optic cup enlarges more extensively in the vertical plane than in the horizontal plane as atrophy progresses. Ischaemic optic atrophy is caused by occlusive disease in the posterior ciliary arteries. The myocilin gene is located on chromosome 1, whereas the optineurin gene is located on the short arm of chromosome 10—both genes have been implicated in the pathogenesis of primary open-angle glaucoma. Myocilin has a role in the contractility of trabecular meshwork cells.

Further reading

Chapter 9: Pathology. In: Forrester JV, Dick AD, McMenamin PG, Roberts F, Pearlman E. *The Eye: Basic Sciences in Practice* (4th Edition). Elsevier (2016).

49. A.

In end-stage Stargardt's disease, the gliotic retina fuses with Bruch's membrane, as the outer retinal layer is lost. On fundoscopy, there are small yellow flecks with a beaten-metal appearance of the macula, due to atrophy of the retinal pigment epithelium. Most cases result from mutations in the *ABCA4* gene. The *SOD2* gene potentially has a role in age-related macular degeneration.

Further reading

Chapter 9: Pathology. In: Forrester JV, Dick AD, McMenamin PG, Roberts F, Pearlman E. *The Eye: Basic Sciences in Practice* (4th Edition). Elsevier (2016).

50. A.

The endothelium and Desçemet's membrane are not involved in granular corneal dystrophy. Non-birefringent hyaline bodies are found in the mid and anterior stroma and Bowman's layer. These stain positively with the Masson trichrome stain (see Table 1.6, p. xxx, and Fig. 1.8, p. xxx). It is inherited in an autosomal dominant manner.

Further reading

Chapter 9: Pathology. In: Forrester JV, Dick AD, McMenamin PG, Roberts F, Pearlman E. *The Eye: Basic Sciences in Practice* (4th Edition). Elsevier (2016).

51. A.

Iris melanomas are typically slow-growing nodular tumours. Uveal melanomas are usually unilateral and initially grow as pigmented/non-pigmented plaque-like lesions. Choroidal melanomas most commonly metastasise to the liver.

Further reading

Chapter 9: Pathology. In: Forrester JV, Dick AD, McMenamin PG, Roberts F, Pearlman E. *The Eye: Basic Sciences in Practice* (4th Edition). Elsevier (2016).

Microbiology

52. B.

Contact lenses represent a major risk factor for corneal infections worldwide. Long-term contact lens wear can inhibit the proliferation and promotion of corneal epithelial cells.

Further reading

Chapter 8: Microbial infections of the eye. In: Forrester JV, Dick AD, McMenamin PG, Roberts F, Pearlman E. *The Eye: Basic Sciences in Practice* (4th Edition). Elsevier (2016).

53. C.

Candida albicans represents the most common yeast responsible for corneal infections. *Aspergillus, Fusarium,* and *Penicillium* are moulds.

Further reading

Chapter 8: Microbial infections of the eye. In: Forrester JV, Dick AD, McMenamin PG, Roberts F, Pearlman E. *The Eye: Basic Sciences in Practice* (4th Edition). Elsevier (2016).

54. B.

Onchocerciasis is also known as river blindness. Live microfilariae cause minimal tissue damage to the eyes and skin. Local death of microfilariae account for almost all associated immunopathology.

Further reading

Chapter 8: Microbial infections of the eye. In: Forrester JV, Dick AD, McMenamin PG, Roberts F, Pearlman E. *The Eye: Basic Sciences in Practice* (4th Edition). Elsevier (2016).

Immunology

55. D.

Monocytes are approximately 12–20 micrometres in size and can feature round, oval, notched, or horseshoe-shaped nuclei. They feature cytoplasm, granules, and mitochondria in abundance. They also possess well-developed Golgi apparatus.

Further reading

Chapter 7: Immunology. In: Forrester JV, Dick AD, McMenamin PG, Roberts F, Pearlman E. *The Eye: Basic Sciences in Practice* (4th Edition). Elsevier (2016).

56. C.

Approximately 50% of patients with acute anterior uveitis are HLA-B27 positive.

Further reading

Chapter 7: Immunology. In: Forrester JV, Dick AD, McMenamin PG, Roberts F, Pearlman E. *The Eye: Basic Sciences in Practice* (4th Edition). Elsevier (2016).

Pharmacology and genetics 2

Pharmacology

57. C.

Estimation of drug clearance from the circulation is a **more** accurate way to assess the efficiency of drug clearance from the circulation as compared to drug half-life.

Further reading

Chapter 6: General and ocular pharmacology. In: Forrester JV, Dick AD, McMenamin PG, Roberts F, Pearlman E. *The Eye: Basic Sciences in Practice* (5th Edition). Elsevier (2021).

58. D.

Nasolacrimal occlusion for 5 minutes restricts the entry of the drug into the nasal cavity and prolongs residence time in the fornix. The use of ointment as a vehicle prolongs the residence time of the drug in the fornix as compared to solution. Ectropion can decrease residence time of the drug in the fornix as it overspills down the cheek—surgical correction can treat this problem. Formulation at acidic or alkaline pH can irritate the eye, causing increased blink rate and lacrimation, thus increasing drug clearance.

Further reading

Chapter 6: General and ocular pharmacology. In: Forrester JV, Dick AD, McMenamin PG, Roberts F, Pearlman E. *The Eye: Basic Sciences in Practice* (5th Edition). Elsevier (2021).

59. D.

Ophthalmic uses of topical antimuscarinic agents, such as cyclopentolate, include cycloplegic refraction and, for patients with iritis, to prevent posterior synechiae (adherence of the iris to the anterior lens capsule). Systemic side effects include dry mouth, sweating, facial flushing, and **tachycardia**. Ocular side effects include conjunctival hyperaemia, blurred vision, photophobia, transient intraocular pressure rise, and even precipitation of acute angle-closure glaucoma.

Further reading

Chapter 6: General and ocular pharmacology. In: Forrester JV, Dick AD, McMenamin PG, Roberts F, Pearlman E. *The Eye: Basic Sciences in Practice* (5th Edition). Elsevier (2021).

60. B.

Photosensitising agents absorb visible and ultraviolet radiation, thereby generating free radicals. Amiodarone **is** a photosensitising agent. Other photosensitising agents include phenothiazines and psoralens.

Further reading

Chapter 6: General and ocular pharmacology. In: Forrester JV, Dick AD, McMenamin PG, Roberts F, Pearlman E. *The Eye: Basic Sciences in Practice* (5th Edition). Elsevier (2021).

61. A.

Acetylcholine represents the major neurotransmitter of the parasympathetic nervous system. Adrenaline, noradrenaline, and acetylcholine all serve as neurotransmitters within the sympathetic nervous system. Adrenaline and noradrenaline are also known as epinephrine and norepinephrine, respectively.

Further reading

Chapter 6: General and ocular pharmacology. In: Forrester JV, Dick AD, McMenamin PG, Roberts F, Pearlman E. *The Eye: Basic Sciences in Practice* (5th Edition). Elsevier (2021).

62. C.

Cetirizine, loratadine, and diphenhydramine act on H_1-receptors. Ranitidine and cimetidine act on H_2-receptors. Ciproxifan acts on H_3-receptors. Thioperamide acts on H_4-receptors.

Further reading

Chapter 6: General and ocular pharmacology. In: Forrester JV, Dick AD, McMenamin PG, Roberts F, Pearlman E. *The Eye: Basic Sciences in Practice* (5th Edition). Elsevier (2021).

Genetics

63. D.

The prophase of the first meiotic division (prophase I) can be subdivided into the following five stages:

1. Leptotene—chromosomes begin to condense.
2. Zygotene—chromosomes pair and form bivalents.

3. Pachytene—main stage of chromosomal thickening.
4. Diplotene—bivalents begin to separate.
5. Diakinesis—bivalents separate and coil tightly.

Further reading

Chapter 3: Genetics. In: Forrester JV, Dick AD, McMenamin PG, Roberts F, Pearlman E. *The Eye: Basic Sciences in Practice* (5th Edition). Elsevier (2021).

64. A.

Aneuploidy results when paired chromosomes fail to disjoin, or is due to delayed movement during **anaphase**. This can result in trisomy (extra chromosome) or monosomy (missing chromosome).

Further reading

Chapter 3: Genetics. In: Forrester JV, Dick AD, McMenamin PG, Roberts F, Pearlman E. *The Eye: Basic Sciences in Practice* (5th Edition). Elsevier (2021).

65. D.

HLA-B27 is strongly associated with ankylosing spondylitis and moderately associated with reactive arthritis. HLA-DR4 is weakly associated with sympathetic ophthalmia and Vogt–Koyanagi–Harada syndrome. HLA-B51 is weakly associated with Behçet syndrome.

Further reading

Chapter 3: Genetics. In: Forrester JV, Dick AD, McMenamin PG, Roberts F, Pearlman E. *The Eye: Basic Sciences in Practice* (5th Edition). Elsevier (2021).

66. D.

OCA2 is associated with oculocutaneous albinism (type 2). *CNGA3* mutation is associated with achromatopsia. *PAX6* mutation is associated with aniridia. *FRMD7* mutation is associated with **idiopathic** infantile nystagmus. All of the above are associated with infantile nystagmus.

Further reading

Chapter 3: Genetics. In: Forrester JV, Dick AD, McMenamin PG, Roberts F, Pearlman E. *The Eye: Basic Sciences in Practice* (5th Edition). Elsevier (2021).

67. B.

Targeting mutation correction can be achieved using the following: ribozymes, which **cleave and repair messenger RNA** (mRNA); anti-sense oligonucleotides, which block mRNA translation; triple helix oligonucleotides, which block gene transcription.

Further reading

Chapter 3: Genetics. In: Forrester JV, Dick AD, McMenamin PG, Roberts F, Pearlman E. *The Eye: Basic Sciences in Practice* (5th Edition). Elsevier (2021).

68. C.

Ubiquitin plays a role in **destroying** phosphorylated cyclins and cyclin inhibitors.

Further reading

Chapter 3: Genetics. In: Forrester JV, Dick AD, McMenamin PG, Roberts F, Pearlman E. *The Eye: Basic Sciences in Practice* (5th Edition). Elsevier (2021).

Investigations 2

69. D.

The Maddox tests are used to assess symptomatic phorias: Maddox **rod** for **distance**, Maddox **wing** for **near**, and **double Maddox rod** for **torsional** phorias. Two Maddox rods are used in the double Maddox rod test: one **red** and one **white**, placed in front of each eye. Distance correction is **required** for the Maddox rod test as the patient must fix on a distant spot of white light. The Maddox rod is positioned **horizontally** for assessment of **horizontal** phorias (red line is seen vertically) and **vertically** for **vertical** phorias (red line is seen horizontally).

Further reading

Denniston AKO, Wolffsohn J, Auld R, Murray PI. Chapter 1: Clinical skills. In: Denniston AKO, Murray PI. *Oxford Handbook of Ophthalmology*. Oxford University Press (2018).

70. C.

The prism cover test is used to measure the angle of deviation. The prism should 'point' towards the direction of deviation. In this case, the prism should be orientated in the base-in position for an exotropia.

Further reading

Denniston AKO, Wolffsohn J, Auld R, Murray PI. Chapter 1: Clinical skills. In: Denniston AKO, Murray PI. *Oxford Handbook of Ophthalmology*. Oxford University Press (2018).

71. D.

The Hirschberg test can detect manifest deviation and simply involves asking the patient to fix on a pen-torch at 33 cm, then assessing the corneal reflection. Normally this should be just nasal to the centre point of the cornea. If the corneal reflection is temporal, the eye is esotropic (convergent), whereas if the reflection is nasal, the eye is exotropic (divergent). 1 mm deviation represents 15 prism dioptres (Δ) or 7°.

Further reading

Denniston AKO, Wolffsohn J, Auld R, Murray PI. Chapter 1: Clinical skills. In: Denniston AKO, Murray PI. *Oxford Handbook of Ophthalmology*. Oxford University Press (2018).

72. B.

Constriction of the peripheral visual fields may occur due to retinal disease such as retinitis pigmentosa, bilateral panretinal photocoagulation, glaucoma, central retinal artery occlusion, papilloedema, bilateral occipital lobe lesions with macular sparing, and functional visual loss (spiralling/crossing of the isopters). Optic nerve coloboma is more likely to cause blind spot enlargement or altitudinal defects.

Further reading

Mollan SP, Calcagni A, Keane PA. Chapter 2: Investigations and their interpretation. In: Denniston AKO, Murray PI. *Oxford Handbook of Ophthalmology*. Oxford University Press (2018).

73. A.

Corneal topography involves curvature mapping across the entire corneal surface. Curvature maps can be constructed by comparing the data with themselves (relative/normalised scales) or against set ranges (absolute scales). Corneal topography can detect macro-irregularities of the cornea, including astigmatism, keratoconus, and pellucid marginal degeneration. Corneal topography was traditionally performed using Placido's disc; modern approaches include scanning slit technology (Orbscan®, Bausch & Lomb) or Scheimpflug imaging (Pentacam®, Oculus), with both systems permitting evaluation of the posterior corneal surface and corneal thickness maps, with greater coverage of the peripheral cornea.

Further reading

Mollan SP, Calcagni A, Keane PA. Chapter 2: Investigations and their interpretation. In: Denniston AKO, Murray PI. *Oxford Handbook of Ophthalmology*. Oxford University Press (2018).

74. D.

Side effects of fundus fluorescein angiography include nausea and vomiting, transient discolouration of skin and urine, pruritis, local irritation/thrombophlebitis due to extravasation of dye at injection site, vasovagal syncope, and anaphylaxis (severe: 1 in 1900; fatal: 1 in 220,000). Side effects of indocyanine green angiography include nausea and vomiting, sneezing and pruritis, staining of stool, backache, vasovagal syncope, and severe anaphylaxis (1 in 1900).

Further reading

Mollan SP, Calcagni A, Keane PA. Chapter 2: Investigations and their interpretation. In: Denniston AKO, Murray PI. *Oxford Handbook of Ophthalmology*. Oxford University Press (2018).

75. B.

The stages of ICG angiography are summarised as follows:

1. Early phase: 2–60 seconds; prominent filling of choroidal arteries.
2. Early mid-phase: 1–3 minutes; increased prominence of choroidal veins.
3. Late mid-phase: 3–15 minutes; diffuse hypofluorescence (due to diffusion of dye from choriocapillaris).
4. Late phase: 15–30 minutes; dye leaves choroidal and retinal circulations but may remain in neovascular tissue.

Further reading

Mollan SP, Calcagni A, Keane PA. Chapter 2: Investigations and their interpretation. In: Denniston AKO, Murray PI. *Oxford Handbook of Ophthalmology*. Oxford University Press (2018).

76. D.

Fig. 1.6 (see p. xxx) displays the layers of the retina on OCT. The correct order of the layers of the retina, from inner (closest to the vitreous) to outer (closest to the choroid), is as follows: **I**nner limiting membrane, **N**erve fibre layer, **G**anglion cell layer, **I**nner plexiform layer, **I**nner nuclear layer, **O**uter plexiform layer, **O**uter nuclear layer, **E**xternal limiting membrane, **E**llipsoid zone, **R**etinal pigment epithelium. A helpful mnemonic to remember this is as follows: **I**n **N**ew **G**eneration, **I**t **I**sn't **O**nly **O**phthalmologists **E**xamining **E**very **R**etina.

Further reading

Mollan SP, Calcagni A, Keane PA. Chapter 2: Investigations and their interpretation. In: Denniston AKO, Murray PI. *Oxford Handbook of Ophthalmology*. Oxford University Press (2018).

77. C.

The following conditions can cause a normal a-wave and reduced scotopic b-wave on ffERG, also termed an 'electronegative' response: X-linked retinoschisis, central retinal artery/vein occlusion (CRAO/CRVO), congenital stationary night blindness (CSNB) (X-linked and autosomal recessive, complete and incomplete forms), quinine toxicity, melanoma-associated retinopathy, and CLN3 (juvenile Batten) disease.

Total retinal detachment and rod-cone dystrophy compromise the photoreceptors and so can cause reduced a-waves and consequently b-waves. Achromatopsia and cone dystrophy can cause abnormal photopic and normal scotopic or dark-adapted ffERGs. Retinitis pigmentosa causes abnormal scotopic and photopic ffERGs (as it also affects cones).

Further reading

Jiang X, Mahroo OA. Negative electroretinograms: genetic and acquired causes, diagnostic approaches and physiological insights. *Eye (Lond)*. 2021 Sep;*35*(9):2419–2437.

78. B.

In the mfERG, numerous small areas of the retina are stimulated with **appropriately scaled** stimuli.

Further reading

Hoffmann MB, Bach M, Kondo M, et al. ISCEV standard for clinical multifocal electroretinography (mfERG) (2021 update). *Documenta Ophthalmologica. Advances in Ophthalmology*. 2021 Feb;*142*(1):5–16.

79. B.

Please see Fig. 1.9 (p. xxx) which displays the normal pattern ERG and pattern VEP waveforms.

Further reading

Mollan SP, Calcagni A, Keane PA. Chapter 2: Investigations and their interpretation. In: Denniston AKO, Murray PI. *Oxford Handbook of Ophthalmology*. Oxford University Press (2018).

Miscellaneous 2

80. C.

The *p*-value is the probability of obtaining the observed data or data that were more extreme due to chance if the null hypothesis (H$_0$) were true. The significance level is denoted by the Greek letter α and conventionally set to 5%. Power = 1 − β where β is the probability of a type II error. A power of at least 80% is considered acceptable in many studies. The effect size is a quantitative measure of the difference between two groups.

Further reading

Bunce C, Patel KV, Xing W, et al. Ophthalmic statistics note 2: absence of evidence is not evidence of absence. *British Journal of Ophthalmology*. 2014;*98*(5):703–705.

81. D.

The STROBE reporting guideline can be used for observational studies in epidemiology (cohort, case–control, and cross-sectional studies). STROBE = Strengthening the Reporting of Observational Studies in Epidemiology. PRISMA = Preferred Reporting Items for Systematic Reviews and Meta-Analyses. CONSORT = Consolidated Standards of Reporting Trials. STARD = Standards for Reporting of Diagnostic accuracy studies. See the EQUATOR Network website for other reporting guidelines with full details.

Further reading

EQUATOR Network. Enhancing the Quality and Transparency of Health Research. Available at: https://www.equator-network.org Accessed October 2021.

82. B.

The **mean** value is the 'average' value, which can be calculated by adding all the data points then dividing by the number of data points. The **median** value is the 'middle' value, which can be found using the following method: (i) order the data points from smallest to largest; (ii) add 1 to the total number of data points then halve this number; (iii) if the result is a whole number, such as 3, then the median value is the 3rd number, whereas if the result is a decimal number, such as 5.5, then the median value lies halfway between the 5th and 6th number (i.e. the average of these two numbers). The **mode** is the most frequently occurring number. In this example, the mean is 54 as per the following calculation:

$$\frac{(32 + 44 + 44 + 74 + 76)}{5} = \frac{270}{5} = 54$$

Further reading

Bunce C, Young-Zvandasara T. Simplified Ophthalmic Statistics (SOS). Part 2: how to summarise your data and why it's a good idea to do so. *Eye News.* 2018;25(2):34–35. Available at: https://www.eyen ews.uk.com/education/trainees/post/sos-simplified-ophthalmic-statistics-part-2-how-to-summarise-your-data-and-why-it-s-a-good-idea-to-do-so Accessed October 2021.

83. D.

In a normally distributed dataset, approximately:

- 68% of values lie within one standard deviation of the mean
- 95% of values lie within two standard deviations of the mean
- 99.7% of values lie within three standard deviations of the mean.

Further reading

Denniston AKO, Moseley M, Murray PI. Chapter 26: Evidence-based ophthalmology. In: Denniston AKO, Murray PI. *Oxford Handbook of Ophthalmology.* Oxford University Press (2018).

84. D.

According to the World Health Organization, at least 2.2 billion people worldwide have a near or distance visual impairment. In at least 1 billion, visual impairment either could have been prevented or is yet to be addressed. The leading causes of visual impairment globally are uncorrected refractive errors, cataract, age-related macular degeneration, glaucoma, diabetic retinopathy, corneal opacity, and trachoma.

Further reading

World Health Organization. Blindness and vision impairment. 14 October 2021. Available at: https://www.who.int/news-room/fact-sheets/detail/blindness-and-visual-impairment Accessed October 2021.

85. B.

Fig. 1.10 (see p. xxx) is a flowchart displaying common statistical tests and rules.

Further reading

Bunce C, Young-Zvandasara T. Simplified Ophthalmic Statistics (SOS). Part 3: which statistical test should I use (if any)? *Eye News.* 2019;25(4):34–36. Available at: https://www.eyenews.uk.com/educat ion/trainees/post/sos-simplified-ophthalmic-statistics-part-3-which-statistical-test-should-i-use-if-any Accessed November 2021.

86. D.

The Pearson correlation coefficient (also known as Pearson's *r* or the Pearson product-moment correlation coefficient) represents a measure of linear correlation between two datasets. Spearman's rank correlation coefficient (also known as Spearman's ρ) represents a non-parametric measure of rank correlation (statistical dependence between the rankings) of two variables. Fig. 1.10 (see p. xxx) is a flowchart displaying common statistical tests and rules.

Further reading

Bunce C, Young-Zvandasara T. Simplified Ophthalmic Statistics (SOS). Part 3: which statistical test should I use (if any)? *Eye News.* 2019;25(4):34–36. Available at: https://www.eyenews.uk.com/educat ion/trainees/post/sos-simplified-ophthalmic-statistics-part-3-which-statistical-test-should-i-use-if-any Accessed November 2021.

87. A.

Lead-time bias occurs when earlier diagnosis of a disease falsely makes it seem like affected patients are surviving longer. Recency bias occurs due to the tendency to favour recent events over older events. Detection bias occurs due to systematic differences between groups in how outcomes are determined. Publication bias is a type of reporting bias, occurring where the outcome of the study influences the decision whether or not to publish it.

Further reading

Denniston AKO, Moseley M, Murray PI. Chapter 26: Evidence-based ophthalmology. In: Denniston AKO, Murray PI. *Oxford Handbook of Ophthalmology.* Oxford University Press (2018).

88.
  I.   D.
  II. C.
  III. C.

Equations for diagnostic accuracy testing:

$$Sensitivity = \frac{TP}{TP + FN}$$

$$Specificity = \frac{TN}{TN + FP}$$

$$PPV = \frac{TP}{TP + FP}$$

$$NPV = \frac{TN}{TN + FN}$$

$$Positive\ likelihood\ ratio = \frac{sensitivity}{1-specificity}$$

$$Negative\ likelihood\ ratio = \frac{1-sensitivity}{specificity}$$

$$Accuracy = \frac{TP+TN}{TP+TN+FP+FN}$$

Further reading

Denniston AKO, Moseley M, Murray PI. Chapter 26: Evidence-based ophthalmology. In: Denniston AKO, Murray PI. *Oxford Handbook of Ophthalmology*. Oxford University Press (2018).

Optics 3

1. **According to the wave theory of light, which of the following best defines wavelength?**
   A. The distance between two symmetrical parts of the wave motion
   B. The maximum displacement of an imaginary particle on the wave from the baseline
   C. Any portion of a cycle
   D. One complete oscillation

2. **Regarding stereopsis, which statement is LEAST likely to be correct?**
   A. Maximum stereoacuity is achieved when images fall on the macula.
   B. Stereoacuity worse than 250 seconds of arc may indicate amblyopia.
   C. Stereopsis is the ability to fuse slightly dissimilar images, which stimulate disparate retinal elements within Panum's areas.
   D. The Wirt fly test is performed at 30 cm and tests a range of stereoacuity from 4000 to 40 seconds of arc.

3. **Regarding prisms, which statement is MOST likely to be correct?**
   A. In the Prentice position, the angle of incidence equals the angle of emergence.
   B. Prism power can be deduced without knowledge of the refractive index of the prism material.
   C. One prism dioptre power produces linear apparent displacement of 1 cm of an object situated at 1 cm.
   D. A Risley prism can be used with a Maddox rod to measure phorias.

4. **Regarding toric lenses, which statement is LEAST likely to be true?**
   A. With respect to the interval of Sturm, the plane where two pencils of light intersect is termed the circle of least confusion.
   B. The focal point of the spherical equivalent coincides with the circle of least confusion, with respect to Sturm's conoid.
   C. Toric lenses do not produce a single defined image.
   D. Toric lenses can be expressed as a fraction where the cylindrical power is the numerator and the spherical power the denominator.

MCQs for FRCOphth Part 1. Sohaib R. Rufai, Oxford University Press. © Oxford University Press 2023.
DOI: 10.1093/oso/9780192843715.003.0003

5. **Regarding measuring lens power, which statement is MOST likely to be correct?**

    A. The Geneva lens measure is calibrated for lenses made of flint glass.
    B. The focimeter can measure the major powers and axes of an astigmatic lens, but not the power of a prism.
    C. With respect to the focimeter, the collimating lens position is fixed but the target can be moved relative to it.
    D. Red light is used during focimetry to eliminate chromatic aberration.

6. **In the reduced eye, what is the distance of the nodal point (N) behind the anterior corneal surface, in millimetres (mm)?**

    A. 1.35 mm
    B. 7.08 mm
    C. −15.7 mm
    D. 24.13 mm

7. **Which of the Purkinje–Sanson images is formed by the anterior lens surface?**

    A. I
    B. II
    C. III
    D. IV

8. **What is the approximate effective power of the crystalline lens *in situ* in an emmetropic eye of normal axial length, in dioptres (D)?**

    A. +15 D
    B. +18 D
    C. +21 D
    D. +24 D

9. **Relative spectacle magnification (RSM) is calculated using which of the following formulae?**

    A. $RSM = \dfrac{uncorrected\ emmetropic\ image\ size}{ametropic\ image\ size}$

    B. $RSM = \dfrac{uncorrected\ ametropic\ image\ size}{emmetropic\ image\ size}$

    C. $RSM = \dfrac{corrected\ emmetropic\ image\ size}{ametropic\ image\ size}$

    D. $RSM = \dfrac{corrected\ ametropic\ image\ size}{emmetropic\ image\ size}$

10. Regarding contact lenses, which of the following forms the tear lens?

A. The tear film covering the inner eyelids

B. The tear film covering the anterior surface of the contact lens and peripheral cornea

C. The tear film covering the conjunctiva

D. The tear film between the anterior surface of the cornea and the posterior surface of the contact lens

11. Regarding the use of the convex lens as a magnifying loupe, which statement is MOST likely to be correct?

A. The standard ×8 loupe possesses a lens power of 16 dioptres

B. The object is situated between the second principal focus and the lens

C. Bar-shaped convex cylindrical lenses used as reading aids produce a horizontal magnification of the letters when placed on a line of printed text

D. The field of vision obtained by a hand or stand magnifier depends on the size of the lens aperture and the eye–lens distance.

12. Regarding direct ophthalmoscopy, which statement is LEAST likely to be true?

A. The field of view is larger when the pupil is dilated, assuming no change in viewing distance.

B. The field of view is smaller in a hypermetropic eye compared to in an emmetropic eye.

C. The field of view is larger when the observer brings the direct ophthalmoscope closer to the patient's eye.

D. The field of view is less than that delivered by the indirect ophthalmoscope.

13. Regarding a zoom lens system, which statement is LEAST likely to be true?

A. In order to magnify an object while keeping the object–lens distance constant, the power of the lens must be varied.

B. The zoom lens system is termed uncompensated if there is a significant change in image position.

C. Several mobile lens elements can be used to achieve a compensated zoom lens system.

D. The fewer lens elements used, the less the image shifts as magnification is varied.

14. Regarding the applanation tonometer, what area of contact in millimetres (mm) is required such that the surface tension and corneal rigidity cancel each other out?

A. 2.86 mm

B. 3.06 mm

C. 3.26 mm

D. 3.46 mm

15. **What radiation wavelength range can enter the eye and reach the retina, in nanometres (nm)?**
    A. 200–1200 nm
    B. 400–1400 nm
    C. 600–1600 nm
    D. 800–1800 nm

16. **Which of the following is LEAST likely to cause glare?**
    A. Corneal oedema
    B. Corneal scarring
    C. Posterior lens capsule opacification
    D. Corneal arcus

Anatomy 3

17. **Which surface of the eyeball is the most exposed?**
    A. Superior
    B. Medial
    C. Inferior
    D. Lateral

18. **Regarding the eyelids, which statement is LEAST likely to be true?**
    A. Each eyelid margin is approximately 2 mm thick
    B. Each eyelid margin is approximately 40 mm long
    C. The papilla lacrimalis is situated approximately 5 mm from the medial angle
    D. The punctum lacrimale is approximately 0.4–0.8 mm in diameter

19. **Regarding the fascial sheath of the eyeball, which statement is LEAST likely to be correct?**
    A. The fascial sheath firmly attaches to the sclera approximately 3 mm posterior to the corneoscleral junction.
    B. All six extraocular muscle tendons pierce the fascial sheath.
    C. The suspensory ligament of Lockwood forms a hammock below the eyeball and between the medial and lateral check ligaments.
    D. The fascial sheath fuses posteriorly with the sclera around the exit of the optic nerve.

20. **What is the distance between the superior rectus muscle and the limbus, in millimetres (mm)?**
    A. 5.5 mm
    B. 6.5 mm
    C. 6.9 mm
    D. 7.7 mm

21. **Regarding the corneal epithelium, which statement is MOST likely to be true?**
    A. The peripheral epithelium is devoid of Langerhans cells.
    B. The total thickness of the epithelium is approximately 50–60 micrometres.
    C. The epithelium becomes continuous with the tarsal conjunctiva at the limbus.
    D. The superficial epithelial cells are columnar while the deepest cells are flattened, nucleated, non-keratinised squamous cells.

22. **Which foramen of the skull perforates the apex of the petrous temporal bone?**
    A. Foramen rotundum
    B. Foramen ovale
    C. Foramen spinosum
    D. Foramen lacerum

23. **Regarding the ciliary body, which statement is MOST likely to be true?**
    A. The ciliary body measures approximately 4 mm wide.
    B. It is cross-sectionally triangular with its base facing the posterior chamber.
    C. Its anterior surface is termed the pars plicata.
    D. Its posterior surface produces aqueous humour.

24. **Regarding the sphincter pupillae, which statement is MOST likely to be true?**
    A. The sphincter pupillae is a ring of smooth muscle measuring approximately 3 mm wide.
    B. The sphincter pupillae is supplied by parasympathetic postganglionic fibres in the long ciliary nerves.
    C. The sphincter pupillae contracts during excitement or fear.
    D. The muscle fibres of the sphincter pupillae are derived from the optic cup.

25. **The inner retina receives its blood supply from the central retinal artery, whereas the outer retina is supplied by the choroidal capillaries. Which retinal layer divides the retina into these inner and outer halves?**
    A. Inner plexiform layer
    B. Inner nuclear layer
    C. Outer plexiform layer
    D. Outer nuclear layer

26. **Regarding the lens, which statement is MOST likely to be true?**
    A. Its anterior surface is more convex than its posterior surface.
    B. Its equator lies approximately 2 mm from the ciliary processes.
    C. Its capsule is thinnest at the anterior pole.
    D. Its anterior suture is an erect 'Y' shape, whereas its posterior suture is an inverted 'Y' shape.

27. **Regarding the extraocular muscles, which statement is MOST likely to be true?**
    A. The muscle fibres are transversely arranged.
    B. The larger diameter fibres occupy the periphery of the muscle.
    C. The lateral rectus possesses the greatest tendon length.
    D. All extraocular muscles arise from the annulus of Zinn.

28. **Regarding the oculomotor nerve, which statement is MOST likely to be correct?**
    A. It emerges from the anterior aspect of the midbrain, lateral to the cerebral peduncle.
    B. It runs forward through the medial wall of the cavernous sinus.
    C. Its superior division terminates at the superior rectus muscle.
    D. The longest branch of its inferior division supplies the inferior oblique muscle.

29. **Which portion of the optic nerve does NOT receive its blood supply from the pial plexus?**
    A. Intraorbital
    B. Intraocular
    C. Intracranial
    D. Intracanalicular

30. **What is the approximate diameter of the eye at the end of the embryonic period (week 8), in millimetres (mm)?**
    A. 0.5–1 mm
    B. 1.5–2 mm
    C. 2.5–3 mm
    D. 3.5–4 mm

Physiology 3

Physiology of the eye and vision

31. **Regarding tear production, which statement is LEAST likely to be true?**
    A. Meibomian glands secrete the lipid layer.
    B. Conjunctival goblet cells secrete mucins.
    C. Cuboidal cells of the corneal and conjunctival epithelium produce the glycocalyx.
    D. The lacrimal gland is the main secretor of the aqueous layer.

32. **Which age group is most likely to display against-the-rule corneal astigmatism?**
    A. 0–20 years
    B. 21–45 years
    C. 46–70 years
    D. 70–90 years

33. **Approximately what percentage volume of the eye is comprised by the vitreous body?**
    A. 50%
    B. 65%
    C. 80%
    D. 95%

34. **In the human fovea, how many photoreceptors interact with one retinal pigment epithelium (RPE) cell, on average?**
    A. 15
    B. 23
    C. 35
    D. 43

35. **Regarding vernier acuity, which statement is LEAST likely to be true?**
    A. Vernier acuity measures the ability to detect a misalignment between two line segments.
    B. Vernier acuity is used to measure distance with a ruler.
    C. Vernier acuity reaches its highest level of function at 8 years of age.
    D. Vernier acuity is absent in strabismic amblyopia.

36. **Approximately how long does regeneration of rhodopsin take in humans, following dark adaptation?**
    A. 15 minutes
    B. 30 minutes
    C. 45 minutes
    D. 60 minutes

General physiology

37. **Regarding anaemia, which statement is LEAST likely to be true?**
    A. Total gastrectomy can result in megaloblastic anaemia.
    B. In hereditary spherocytosis, the red blood cells cannot withstand compression forces.
    C. Haemoglobin S contains faulty alpha chains in the haemoglobin molecule.
    D. In erythroblastosis fetalis, antibodies from the rhesus-negative mother attack rhesus-positive red blood cells in the fetus.

38. **Regarding the electrocardiogram (ECG), which statement is MOST likely to be true?**
    A. The P wave represents atrial repolarisation.
    B. The T wave represents ventricular depolarisation.
    C. The PR interval is normally 0.16 seconds.
    D. The QT interval is normally approximately 0.5 seconds.

39. **Regarding pulmonary volumes in the average adult male in millilitres (mL), which statement is LEAST likely to be correct?**
    A. Inspiratory reserve volume is 1500 mL.
    B. Expiratory reserve volume is 1100 mL.
    C. Tidal volume is 500 mL.
    D. Residual volume is 1200 mL.

40. **Which of the following chemicals CANNOT directly excite pain receptors?**
    A. Bradykinin
    B. Prostaglandins
    C. Serotonin
    D. Potassium ions

41. **Regarding the nephron, which statement is MOST likely to be true?**
    A. Each human kidney contains approximately 100,000 nephrons.
    B. Juxtamedullary nephrons comprise 20–30% of all nephrons.
    C. Cortical nephrons have longer loops of Henle than juxtamedullary nephrons.
    D. The collecting duct becomes impermeable to water in the presence of antidiuretic hormone.

Biochemistry

42. **Approximately what percentage of the tear film is comprised by the aqueous layer?**
    A. 95%
    B. 80%
    C. 60%
    D. 40%

43. **Regarding the vascular function of the choroid, which statement is LEAST likely to be true?**
    A. Of the blood supplied to the eye, approximately 98% passes through the uveal tract, 85% of which is via the choroid.
    B. Blood flow via the choroid takes place at a rate of 1400 millilitres/minute per 100 grams of tissue.
    C. The choriocapillaris possess a lobular architecture.
    D. Choroidal blood vessels are not fenestrated.

Pathology 3

General and ocular pathology

44. Regarding vasculitides, which statement is MOST likely to be true?

A. Giant cell arteritis and Takayasu's disease usually occur in individuals over 50 years of age.

B. Giant cell arteritis involves the cerebral arteries, ophthalmic arteries, anterior ciliary branches, and central retinal arteries.

C. Polyarteritis nodosa and Kawasaki disease affect medium-sized blood vessels.

D. Granulomatosis with polyangiitis is a large-vessel vasculitis causing granulomatous inflammation and necrosis.

45. Regarding basal cell carcinoma (BCC), which statement is LEAST likely to be correct?

A. It accounts for 90% of malignant eyelid tumours.

B. It can occur in association with Gorlin–Goltz syndrome in younger individuals.

C. Superficial and nodular growth patterns are associated with a high risk of recurrence.

D. They can be associated with a malignant squamous component.

46. Regarding the polymerase chain reaction (PCR), which statement is MOST likely to be true?

A. The three steps of PCR are carried out in the following order: denaturation, extension, and annealing.

B. Denaturation is followed by annealing of synthetic oligonucleotide primers, specifically designed to separate the target nucleic acid region.

C. During a typical PCR analysis, 10–20 cycles are carried out.

D. Denaturation of the target nucleic acid renders it single stranded.

47. Regarding herpes zoster virus, which statement is LEAST likely to be true?

A. The virus can infect the ganglia and branches of the trigeminal nerve.

B. When reactivated, the virus can replicate and produce skin vesicles in the distribution of the affected nerve or branches thereof.

C. In herpes zoster ophthalmicus, the inflammatory process can involve the uveal tract, cornea, conjunctiva, and eyelids.

D. A monocytic infiltrate typically appears around the long and short ciliary nerves in herpes zoster ophthalmicus.

48. Regarding primary closed-angle glaucoma, which statement is LEAST likely to be true?

A. The lens thickens anteroposteriorly with age.

B. Pressure build-up behind the iris pushes the peripheral iris towards the trabecular meshwork.

C. Papilloedema is secondary to the blockage of axoplasmic flow.

D. The anterior lens surface displaces the peripheral zone of the iris anteriorly.

49. **Which of the following corneal dystrophies is inherited in an autosomal recessive manner?**
   A. Reis–Bücklers dystrophy
   B. Lattice dystrophy
   C. Macular dystrophy
   D. Granular dystrophy

50. **Regarding acute retinal necrosis, which statement is LEAST likely to be true?**
   A. This condition usually occurs in immunocompromised individuals.
   B. The most common causes are infection with varicella zoster or herpes simplex virus.
   C. Light microscopy can reveal intranuclear viral inclusion bodies.
   D. The dimension of the infective viral particle ranges from 190 nanometres to 220 nanometres.

51. **Which of the following is associated with a MORE favourable diagnosis in patients with uveal melanoma?**
   A. Ciliary body location
   B. Closed loop vascular pattern revealed on periodic acid–Schiff stain
   C. Epithelioid cell component
   D. Numerical gain of chromosome 6p

Microbiology

52. **Which of the following adenovirus serotypes is LEAST likely to cause epidemic keratoconjunctivitis?**
   A. 3
   B. 7
   C. 14
   D. 19

53. **Regarding *Pseudomonas aeruginosa*, which statement is LEAST likely to be true?**
   A. It is a Gram-negative bacillus.
   B. It is ubiquitous in fresh water.
   C. It is the second most common cause of bacterial keratitis globally.
   D. Corneal injury and contact lens wear are major risk factors for *Pseudomonas aeruginosa* keratitis.

54. **Regarding *Aspergillus* keratitis, which statement is LEAST likely to be true?**
   A. Conidia are produced on conidiophores and dispersed by wind.
   B. Hyphal tips contain collagenases, which permit migration throughout the corneal stroma.
   C. Topical natamycin can be effective in treating *Aspergillus* keratitis if administered early.
   D. If treatment is delayed, hyphae can penetrate into the posterior segment.

Immunology

55. Regarding the innate immune system and the eye, which statement is LEAST likely to be true?

A. The conjunctiva contains dendritic cells.

B. Tear lipid possesses an antibacterial effect, applying to both short-chain and long-chain fatty acids.

C. Lysozyme is effective against Gram-positive organisms.

D. Polymorphonuclear leucocytes in the tears increase in number during sleep.

56. Regarding Stevens–Johnson syndrome, which statement is LEAST likely to be true?

A. Subconjunctival fibrosis occurs in Stevens–Jonson syndrome.

B. The drug acts as a hapten.

C. Stevens–Jonson syndrome is self-limiting.

D. The severity of the condition is unrelated by the duration of exposure to the causative drug.

Pharmacology and genetics 3

Pharmacology

57. Regarding receptors, which statement is LEAST likely to be true?

A. A ligand is a drug or natural substance that binds to a receptor.

B. An agonist is a substance that results in stimulation or inhibition of cell function, when bound to a receptor.

C. A partial agonist has a higher maximal effect than a pure agonist.

D. An antagonist is a substance that prevents the activation of a receptor.

58. Which of the following classes of topically applied drugs lower intraocular pressure mainly by increasing uveoscleral outflow of aqueous humour?

A. β-blockers

B. Carbonic anhydrase inhibitors

C. Parasympathomimetics

D. Prostaglandin analogues

59. Which of the following is LEAST likely to be a systemic side effect of topical β-blockers?

A. Facial flushing

B. Bradycardia

C. Syncope

D. Bronchospasm

60. Which of the following immunosuppressants acts on cytosolic receptors and blocks the transcription of cytokine genes?

A. Ciclosporin
B. Tacrolimus
C. Azathioprine
D. Corticosteroids

61. Which adrenergic receptors relax the smooth muscle of blood vessels and bronchi?

A. α_1
B. α_2
C. β_1
D. β_2

62. Which histamine receptor does ciproxifan act on?

A. H_1
B. H_2
C. H_3
D. H_4

Genetics

63. Regarding molecular genetics, which statement is MOST likely to be true?

A. The human haploid genome comprises 3×10^9 base pairs of single-stranded DNA.
B. Tryptophan can only be encoded by one codon, TGG.
C. Methionine can be encoded by more than one codon.
D. Introns are coding regions of a gene.

64. Regarding structural chromosomal abnormalities, which statement is LEAST likely to be true?

A. Point mutations can alter amino acid coding.
B. Insertional translocation requires three breaks in one or two chromosomes.
C. Translocation does not typically cause loss of DNA.
D. Inversions occur following two chromosomal breaks, where the segment is inverted 90° between the two breaks.

65. Human leukocyte antigen (HLA)-B27 is MOST strongly associated with which of the following conditions?

A. Reactive arthritis
B. Ankylosing spondylitis
C. Behçet syndrome
D. Acute anterior uveitis

66. **Which of the following gene mutations is NOT associated with congenital glaucoma or juvenile open-angle glaucoma?**
    A. *OPTN*
    B. *GPR179*
    C. *MYOC*
    D. *CYP1B1*

67. **Regarding vectors, which statement is LEAST likely to be true?**
    A. Adenoviruses can be programmed to remove antigenic coats.
    B. Retroviruses possess reverse transcriptase.
    C. Liposomes can efficiently transport DNA of any size.
    D. Adeno-associated viruses can only carry smaller DNA inserts but can achieve long-term expression.

68. **Which of the following gene mutations is responsible for congenital stationary night blindness?**
    A. *PITX2*
    B. *NYX*
    C. *OPA1*
    D. *TIMP3*

Investigations 3

69. **Regarding assessment of binocular status, which test uses polaroid glasses?**
    A. Lang
    B. TNO
    C. Frisby
    D. Titmus

70. **Regarding the Maddox rod test where a single Maddox rod is placed horizontally in front of the right eye fixing on a white light, what is indicated by the line appearing to the left of the white light?**
    A. Right esophoria
    B. Right exophoria
    C. Left esophoria
    D. Left exophoria

71. **Which of the following visual field defects is MOST likely to be caused by tilted disc syndrome?**
    A. Bitemporal hemianopia
    B. Homonymous hemianopia
    C. Binasal field defect
    D. Altitudinal field defect

72. **Regarding anterior segment imaging, which statement is LEAST likely to be true?**
    A. Optical coherence tomography (OCT) permits visualisation of the iridocorneal angle.
    B. *In vivo* confocal microscopy uses pinhole apertures conjugate to the focal plane.
    C. Anterior segment OCT uses shorter-wavelength light than posterior segment OCT.
    D. *In vivo* confocal microscopy can be used to evaluate filtering blebs post-trabeculectomy.

73. **What is the correct order of the phases of fundus fluorescein angiography?**
    A. Choroidal, arterial, capillary, venous, late
    B. Choroidal, venous, arterial, capillary, late
    C. Choroidal, arterial, venous, capillary, late
    D. Choroidal, venous, capillary, arterial, late

74. **In indocyanine green (ICG) angiography, which of the following is MOST likely to cause a filling defect?**
    A. Choroidal neovascularisation
    B. Choroidal haemangioma
    C. Atrophic age-related macular degeneration
    D. Retinal pigment epithelium defect

75. **What is the layer marked with an arrow on this optical coherence tomography (OCT) image?**

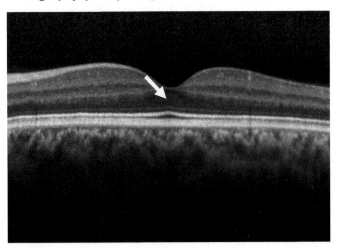

    A. Inner nuclear layer
    B. Outer nuclear layer
    C. Ganglion cell layer
    D. External limiting membrane

76. **Which of the following is LEAST likely to represent an indication for ocular ultrasonography?**
    A. Axial length measurement
    B. Detection of posterior segment pathology
    C. Anterior chamber depth measurement
    D. Assessment of thyroid eye disease

77. **Regarding ultrasound biomicroscopy (UBM), which statement is LEAST likely to be true?**
    A. It permits less depth penetration than standard ocular ultrasonography.
    B. It uses a lower frequency transducer than standard ocular ultrasonography.
    C. It delivers higher resolution than standard ocular ultrasonography.
    D. It can be used to evaluate anterior segment tumours.

78. **Which electrophysiological test would be MOST appropriate to exclude hydroxychloroquine toxicity?**
    A. Multifocal electroretinogram
    B. Electro-oculogram
    C. Pattern visual evoked potential
    D. Flash visual evoked potential

79. **Regarding the electro-oculogram (EOG), which statement is LEAST likely to be true?**
    A. It measures the standing potential at the retinal pigment epithelium–photoreceptor interface.
    B. Electrodes are positioned at the medial and lateral canthi.
    C. The patient intermittently follows targets moving right to left over a 60° horizontal plane.
    D. The result is a ratio of light peak:dark trough

Miscellaneous 3

80. **Which of the following best defines the statistical term 'sensitivity'?**
    A. The proportion of people with a positive test who have the disease.
    B. The proportion of healthy people who test negative.
    C. The proportion of diseased people who test positive.
    D. The proportion of people with a negative test who are healthy.

81. **For which study type should the CONSORT reporting guideline be used?**
    A. Diagnostic accuracy study
    B. Case–control study
    C. Systematic review
    D. Randomised controlled trial

82. **What is the median value of the following numbers?**

    33, 28, 14, 19, 17, 42, 7, 11, 16, 22

    A. 16
    B. 17
    C. 18
    D. 19

83. **In a normally distributed dataset, approximately what percentage of values lie within two standard deviations of the mean?**

    A. 90%
    B. 93%
    C. 95%
    D. 99%

84. **Which of the following statements does NOT represent one of Wilson and Junger's ten principles for a good screening test?**

    A. The natural history of the condition, including development from latent to declared disease, should be adequately understood.
    B. There should be a recognisable latent or early symptomatic phase.
    C. The cost of case-finding (including a diagnosis and treatment of patients diagnosed) should be economically balanced in relation to possible expenditure on medical care as a whole.
    D. There should be a 'once and for all' project.

85. **What is the MOST appropriate statistical test to use for three groups where the outcome measure is continuous and the data are parametric?**

    A. Unpaired t-test
    B. Kruskal–Wallis test
    C. Analysis of variance
    D. Mann–Whitney U test

86. **Regarding the Wilcoxon signed rank test, which statement is MOST likely to be correct?**

    A. It should be used when the outcome measure is continuous and the data are parametric and paired.
    B. It should be used when the outcome measure is continuous and the data are non-parametric and unpaired.
    C. It should be used when the outcome measure is continuous and the data are non-parametric and paired.
    D. It should be used when the outcome measure is categorical and the data are unpaired.

87. **Which of the following options represents the MOST likely cause of detection bias?**

    A. The tendency to favour recent events over older events
    B. Earlier diagnosis of a disease falsely makes it seem like affected patients are surviving longer
    C. The outcome of the study influences the decision whether or not to publish it
    D. Systematic differences between groups in how outcomes are determined

88. **A team of researchers have developed a new test to detect primary open-angle glaucoma (POAG). Their study results are displayed in the following 2 × 2 table:**

	POAG present	POAG absent
Index test positive	80	10
Index test negative	20	90

    I.   What is the sensitivity of the new test to detect POAG, in per cent and to the nearest whole number?
        A. 80%
        B. 82%
        C. 85%
        D. 90%
    II. What is the specificity of the new test to detect POAG, in per cent and to the nearest whole number?
        A. 80%
        B. 82%
        C. 85%
        D. 90%
    III. What is the negative predictive value of the new test to detect POAG, in per cent and to the nearest whole number?
        A. 80%
        B. 82%
        C. 85%
        D. 90%

Optics 3

1. A.

The wavelength is the distance between two symmetrical parts of the wave motion, i.e. the distance over which the wave's shape repeats. Amplitude is the maximum displacement of an imaginary particle on the wave from the baseline. Phase is any portion of a cycle. The cycle is one complete oscillation.

Further reading

Chapter 1: Properties of light and visual function. In: Elkington AR, Frank HJ, Greaney MJ. *Clinical Optics*. Blackwell Science (1999).

2. D.

The Wirt fly test is performed at 40 cm and tests a range of stereoacuity from 3000 to 40 seconds of arc. Other responses are true.

Further reading

Chapter 1: Properties of light and visual function. In: Elkington AR, Frank HJ, Greaney MJ. *Clinical Optics*. Blackwell Science (1999).

3. D.

In the Prentice position, the angle of incidence does **not** equal the angle of emergence. The prism power **cannot** be deduced without knowledge of the refractive index of the prism material. One prism dioptre power produces linear apparent displacement of 1 cm of an object situated at 1 m (not cm).

Further reading

Chapter 4: Prisms. In: Elkington AR, Frank HJ, Greaney MJ. *Clinical Optics*. Blackwell Science (1999).

4. D.

Toric lenses can be expressed as a fraction where the spherical power is the numerator and the cylindrical power the denominator. Other options are true.

Further reading

Chapter 6: Astigmatic lenses. In: Elkington AR, Frank HJ, Greaney MJ. *Clinical Optics*. Blackwell Science (1999).

5. C.

The Geneva lens measure is calibrated for lenses made of crown glass. The focimeter can measure the major powers and axes of an astigmatic lens and the power of a prism. Green light is used during focimetry to eliminate chromatic aberration.

Further reading

Chapter 7: Optical prescriptions, spectacle lenses. In: Elkington AR, Frank HJ, Greaney MJ. *Clinical Optics*. Blackwell Science (1999).

6. B.

A = principal point (P); C = first focal point; D = second focal point. See Fig. 1.4 (p. xxx) for a schematic of the reduced eye schematic and Table 1.3 (p. xxx) for distances of cardinal points behind the anterior corneal surface as per the reduced eye.

Further reading

Chapter 9: Refraction by the eye. In: Elkington AR, Frank HJ, Greaney MJ. *Clinical Optics*. Blackwell Science (1999).

7. C.

Images I and II are formed from the anterior and posterior corneal surfaces, respectively. Images III and IV are formed from the anterior and posterior lens surfaces, respectively.

Further reading

Chapter 9: Refraction by the eye. In: Elkington AR, Frank HJ, Greaney MJ. *Clinical Optics*. Blackwell Science (1999).

8. A.

The effective power of the crystalline lens *in situ* is +15 D. However, in order to achieve −15 D correction in the plane of the crystalline lens, due to the increased distance and reduced effectivity of lenses, a spectacle correction of approximately −18 D to −20 D would be required.

Further reading

Chapter 10: Optics of ametropia. In: Elkington AR, Frank HJ, Greaney MJ. *Clinical Optics*. Blackwell Science (1999).

9. D.

Spectacle magnification is the ratio between corrected image size and uncorrected image size. RSM is the ratio between corrected ametropic image size and emmetropic image size.

Further reading

Chapter 10: Optics of ametropia. In: Elkington AR, Frank HJ, Greaney MJ. *Clinical Optics*. Blackwell Science (1999).

10. D.

The tear lens is an optical lens comprising the tear film between the anterior surface of the cornea and posterior surface of the contact lens. In rigid contact lenses, the power of the tear lens varies depending on the shape of the lens and cornea. In soft contact lenses, or if the tear lens possesses uniform thickness, the tear lens has plano power.

Further reading

Chapter 12: Contact lenses. In: Elkington AR, Frank HJ, Greaney MJ. *Clinical Optics*. Blackwell Science (1999).

11. D.

The standard ×8 possesses a lens power of 32 dioptres. The object is situated between the first principal focus and the lens. Bar-shaped convex cylindrical lenses used as reading aids produce a vertical magnification of the letters when placed on a line of printed text.

Further reading

Chapter 13: Optics of low vision aids. In: Elkington AR, Frank HJ, Greaney MJ. *Clinical Optics*. Blackwell Science (1999).

12. B.

The field of view is larger in a hypermetropic eye compared to an emmetropic eye, and smaller in a myopic eye compared to an emmetropic eye.

Further reading

Chapter 14: Instruments. In: Elkington AR, Frank HJ, Greaney MJ. *Clinical Optics*. Blackwell Science (1999).

13. D.

Generally speaking, the more lens elements used, the less the image shifts as magnification is varied.

Further reading

Chapter 14: Instruments. In: Elkington AR, Frank HJ, Greaney MJ. *Clinical Optics*. Blackwell Science (1999).

14. B.

When the area of contact is 3.06 mm, the surface tension and corneal rigidity cancel each other out and the force of application of the tonometer is proportional to the intraocular pressure. See Fig. 2.5 (p. xxx) showing a schematic displaying the appearance of the semicircles viewed using the Goldmann applanation tonometer when the area is too small, correct and too large.

Further reading

Chapter 14: Instruments. In: Elkington AR, Frank HJ, Greaney MJ. *Clinical Optics*. Blackwell Science (1999).

15. B.

Radiation wavelengths ranging from 400 nm to 1400 nm can enter the eye and reach the retina. The effects can be thermal, photochemical, or ionising, depending on the absorption characteristics of the target tissue and the wavelength and pulse duration of the laser light.

Further reading

Chapter 15: Lasers. In: Elkington AR, Frank HJ, Greaney MJ. *Clinical Optics*. Blackwell Science (1999).

16. D.

Corneal arcus results from phospholipid and cholesterol deposits in the peripheral corneal stroma, which can appear as a whitish-grey or blue ring. Options A–C are most likely to cause glare.

Further reading

Chapter 1: Properties of light and visual function. In: Elkington AR, Frank HJ, Greaney MJ. *Clinical Optics*. Blackwell Science (1999).

Chapter 7: Cornea. In: Denniston AKO, Murray PI. *Oxford Handbook of Ophthalmology*. Oxford University Press (2018).

Anatomy 3

17. D.

The lateral surface of the eyeball is the most exposed, as the lateral orbital margin is the least prominent.

Further reading

Chapter 6: The eyeball. In: Snell RS, Lemp MA. *Clinical Anatomy of the Eye* (2nd Edition). John Wiley and Sons (1998).

18. B.

Each eyelid margin is approximately 30 mm long. Other responses are true.

Further reading

Chapter 3: The orbital cavity. In: Snell RS, Lemp MA. *Clinical Anatomy of the Eye* (2nd Edition). John Wiley and Sons (1998).

19. A.

The fascial sheath firmly attaches to the sclera approximately 1.5 mm posterior to the corneoscleral junction. The suspensory ligament of Lockwood is made up of a blending of the sheath of the inferior oblique and inferior rectus muscles.

Further reading

Chapter 6: The eyeball. In: Snell RS, Lemp MA. *Clinical Anatomy of the Eye* (2nd Edition). John Wiley and Sons (1998).

20. D.

The distance between the recti insertions and limbus are as follows: **M**edial, 5.5 mm; **I**nferior, 6.5 mm; **L**ateral: 6.9 mm; **S**uperior: 7.7 mm. You can remember the order using the acronym **MILS**. These insertions form an imaginary spiral called the spiral of Tillaux (see Fig. 2.6, p. xxx). Please note that different textbooks quote slightly different measurements.

Further reading

Chapter 6: The eyeball. In: Snell RS, Lemp MA. *Clinical Anatomy of the Eye* (2nd Edition). John Wiley and Sons (1998).

21. B.

Langerhans cells (immunocompetent dendritic cells) are present in the peripheral corneal epithelium but typically absent in the central epithelium. The epithelium becomes continuous with the bulbar conjunctiva at the limbus. The superficial epithelial cells are flattened, nucleated, non-keratinised squamous cells while the deepest cells are columnar.

Further reading

Chapter 6: The eyeball. In: Snell RS, Lemp MA. *Clinical Anatomy of the Eye* (2nd Edition). John Wiley and Sons (1998).

22. D.

The foramen lacerum perforates the apex of the petrous temporal bone, whereas the foramen rotundum, foramen ovale, and foramen spinosum perforate the greater wing of sphenoid.

Further reading

Chapter 1: An overview of the anatomy of the skull. In: Snell RS, Lemp MA. *Clinical Anatomy of the Eye* (2nd Edition). John Wiley and Sons (1998).

Chapter 1: Anatomy of the eye and orbit. In: Forrester JV, Dick AD, McMenamin PG, Roberts F, Pearlman E. *The Eye: Basic Sciences in Practice* (4th Edition). Elsevier (2016).

23. C.

The ciliary body measures approximately 6 mm wide (6.5 mm temporally and 5.5 mm nasally). It is cross-sectionally triangular with its base facing the anterior chamber. Its anterior surface produces aqueous humour.

Further reading

Chapter 6: The eyeball. In: Snell RS, Lemp MA. *Clinical Anatomy of the Eye* (2nd Edition). John Wiley and Sons (1998).

24. D.

The sphincter pupillae is a ring of smooth muscle measuring approximately 1 mm wide. It is supplied by parasympathetic postganglionic fibres in the short ciliary nerves. The dilator pupillae contracts and dilates the pupil during excitement or fear and in low-intensity light.

Further reading

Chapter 6: The eyeball. In: Snell RS, Lemp MA. *Clinical Anatomy of the Eye* (2nd Edition). John Wiley and Sons (1998).

25. C.

The outer plexiform layer divides the retina into the inner and outer halves supplied by the central retinal artery and choroidal capillaries, respectively. The choroidal capillaries are derived from the ciliary vasculature. Fig. 1.6 (see p. xxx) displays the layers of the retina as seen on optical coherence tomography.

Further reading

Chapter 6: The eyeball. In: Snell RS, Lemp MA. *Clinical Anatomy of the Eye* (2nd Edition). John Wiley and Sons (1998).

26. D.

Its posterior surface is more convex than its anterior surface. Its equator lies approximately 0.5 mm from the ciliary processes. Its capsule is thickest on its anterior and posterior surfaces near the equator (approximately 20 micrometres) and thinnest at the posterior pole (approximately 3 micrometres). Please note that these values vary between sources.

Further reading

Chapter 6: The eyeball. In: Snell RS, Lemp MA. *Clinical Anatomy of the Eye* (2nd Edition). John Wiley and Sons (1998).

27. C.

The extraocular muscle fibres are longitudinally arranged. The larger diameter fibres occupy the centre of the muscle, thereby forming its bulk, whereas the smaller diameter fibres typically occupy the periphery. The four rectus muscles arise from the common tendinous ring, also known as the annulus of Zinn, whereas the superior oblique originates on the body of sphenoid superomedial to the optic canal, while the inferior oblique originates from the orbital floor posterior to the orbital margin and lateral to the nasolacrimal canal.

Further reading

Chapter 1: Anatomy of the eye and orbit. In: Forrester JV, Dick AD, McMenamin PG, Roberts F, Pearlman E. *The Eye: Basic Sciences in Practice* (4th Edition). Elsevier (2016).

Chapter 8: Movements of the eyeball and the extraocular muscles. In: Snell RS, Lemp MA. *Clinical Anatomy of the Eye* (2nd Edition). John Wiley and Sons (1998).

28. D.

The oculomotor nerve, entirely motor in function, emerges from the anterior aspect of the midbrain, medial to the cerebral peduncle. It runs through the lateral wall of the cavernous sinus (Fig. 3.1). Its superior division terminates by supplying the levator palpebrae superioris muscle, after having supplied the superior rectus muscle.

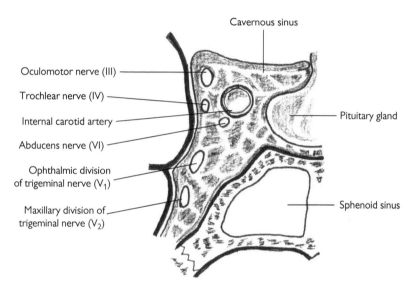

Figure 3.1 The cavernous sinus.

Figure courtesy of Mr Syed Riyaz Ahmad, retired ophthalmologist, Essex, UK.

Further reading

Chapter 10: Cranial nerves—part 1: the nerves directly associated with the eye and orbit. In: Snell RS, Lemp MA. *Clinical Anatomy of the Eye* (2nd Edition). John Wiley and Sons (1998).

29. B.

The intraocular portion of the optic nerve receives its blood supply from branches of the anastomotic circle of Zinn, which is supplied by the short posterior ciliary arteries.

Further reading

Chapter 13: The visual pathway. In: Snell RS, Lemp MA. *Clinical Anatomy of the Eye* (2nd Edition). John Wiley and Sons (1998).

30. B.

At the end of the embryonic period, defined as the end of week 8, the eye is approximately 1.5–2 mm in diameter.

Further reading

Chapter 1: Anatomy of the eye and orbit. In: Forrester JV, Dick AD, McMenamin PG, Roberts F, Pearlman E. *The Eye: Basic Sciences in Practice* (4th Edition). Elsevier (2016).

Physiology 3

Physiology of the eye and vision

31. C.

Stratified squamous cells of the corneal and conjunctival epithelium produce the glycocalyx.

Further reading

Dartt DA. Chapter 15: Formation and function of the tear film. In: Levin LA, Nilsson SFE, Ver Hoeve J, et al. *Adler's Physiology of the Eye* (11th Edition). Elsevier (2011).

32. D.

With-the-rule corneal astigmatism occurs when the vertical meridian is steeper than the horizontal—this is more common in children. Against-the-rule astigmatism occurs when the horizontal meridian is steeper than the vertical—this occurs with ageing and is more common among the elderly.

Further reading

Dawson DG, Ubels JL, Edelhauser HF. Chapter 4: Cornea and sclera. In: Levin LA, Nilsson SFE, Ver Hoeve J, et al. *Adler's Physiology of the Eye* (11th Edition). Elsevier (2011).

33. C.

Approximately 80% of the volume of the eye is comprised by the vitreous body, making it the largest single structure within the eye.

Further reading

Lund-Anderson H, Sander B. Chapter 6: The vitreous. In: Levin LA, Nilsson SFE, Ver Hoeve J, et al. *Adler's Physiology of the Eye* (11th Edition). Elsevier (2011).

34. B.

In the human fovea, each RPE cell interacts with a mean of 23 photoreceptors.

Further reading

Strauss O, Helbig H. Chapter 13: The function of the retinal pigment epithelium. In: Levin LA, Nilsson SFE, Ver Hoeve J, et al. *Adler's Physiology of the Eye* (11th Edition). Elsevier (2011).

35. C.

Vernier acuity reaches its highest level of function at approximately 14 years of age. It may be present in anisometropic amblyopia.

Further reading

Chapter 5: Physiology of vision and the visual system. In: Forrester JV, Dick AD, McMenamin PG, Roberts F, Pearlman E. *The Eye: Basic Sciences in Practice* (4th Edition). Elsevier (2016).

36. B.

Following dark adaptation, regeneration of rhodopsin in humans takes approximately 30 minutes.

Further reading

Chapter 5: Physiology of vision and the visual system. In: Forrester JV, Dick AD, McMenamin PG, Roberts F, Pearlman E. *The Eye: Basic Sciences in Practice* (4th Edition). Elsevier (2016).

General physiology

37. C.

Normal red blood cells possess a biconcave disc shape, permitting the cells to deform and travel through capillaries. In sickle cell anaemia, the abnormal haemoglobin S contains faulty beta chains in the haemoglobin molecule. Low oxygen tension promotes red blood cell sickling. The cell membrane becomes rigid and highly fragile, resulting in haemolysis and serious anaemia.

Further reading

Chapter 33: Red blood cells, anemia, and polycythemia. In: Hall JE. *Guyton and Hall Textbook of Medical Physiology* (13th Edition). Elsevier (2016).

38. C.

The P wave represents atrial depolarisation. The QRS complex represents ventricular repolorisation. The T wave represents ventricular repolarisation. The PR interval is normally 0.16 seconds. The QT interval is normally approximately 0.35 seconds. Fig. 3.2 summarises the ECG waveform in normal sinus rhythm.

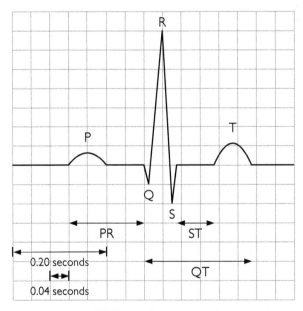

Figure 3.2 The electrocardiogram (ECG) waveform in normal sinus rhythm.

Figure courtesy of Mr Umar Ahmed, Medical Student, Imperial College London.

Further reading

Chapter 11: The normal electrocardiogram. In: Hall JE. *Guyton and Hall Textbook of Medical Physiology* (13th Edition). Elsevier (2016).

39. A.

Inspiratory reserve volume is approximately 3000 mL in the average adult male. Tidal volume is the volume of air inspired/expired in a normal breath. Inspiratory/expiratory reserve volume is that which can be inspired/expired with full force, over and above normal tidal volume. Residual volume represents the remaining volume of air in the lungs following expiration with full force.

Further reading

Chapter 38: Pulmonary ventilation. In: Hall JE. *Guyton and Hall Textbook of Medical Physiology* (13th Edition). Elsevier (2016).

40. B.

Prostaglandins and substance P cannot directly excite pain receptors, rather than merely enhance their sensitivity. Bradykinin, serotonin, histamine, acetylcholine, acids, potassium ions, and proteolytic enzymes can all directly excite pain receptors.

Further reading

Chapter 49: Somatic sensations: II. Pain, headache and thermal sensations. In: Hall JE. *Guyton and Hall Textbook of Medical Physiology* (13th Edition). Elsevier (2016).

41. B.

Each human kidney contains approximately **800,000 to 1 million nephrons**. Cortical nephrons have **shorter** loops of Henle than juxtamedullary nephrons. The collecting duct becomes **permeable** to water in the presence of antidiuretic hormone.

Further reading

Chapter 26: The urinary system: functional anatomy and urine formation by the kidneys. In: Hall JE. *Guyton and Hall Textbook of Medical Physiology* (13th Edition). Elsevier (2016).

Biochemistry

42. C.

The aqueous layer comprises approximately 60% of the tear film.

Further reading

Chapter 4: Biochemistry and cell biology. In: Forrester JV, Dick AD, McMenamin PG, Roberts F, Pearlman E. *The Eye: Basic Sciences in Practice* (5th Edition). Elsevier (2021).

43. D.

Choroidal blood vessels are highly fenestrated and leaky, akin to the ciliary blood vessels.

Further reading

Chapter 4: Biochemistry and cell biology. In: Forrester JV, Dick AD, McMenamin PG, Roberts F, Pearlman E. *The Eye: Basic Sciences in Practice* (5th Edition). Elsevier (2021).

Pathology 3

General and ocular pathology

44. C.

Giant cell arteritis usually occurs in individuals over 50 years of age, whereas Takayasu's disease usually occurs in individuals under 50 years of age. Giant cell arteritis involves the cerebral arteries, ophthalmic arteries, posterior ciliary branches (not the anterior ciliary branches), and central retinal arteries. Granulomatosis with polyangiitis is a small-vessel vasculitis causing granulomatous inflammation and necrosis. Fig. 3.3 displays histopathological slides for a normal temporal artery and temporal arteritis.

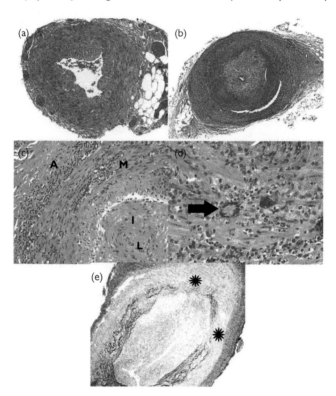

Figure 3.3 Histopathological slides displaying a normal temporal artery and temporal arteritis. (a) Haematoxylin and eosin (H&E) stain of a normal temporal artery (which is an example of a muscular artery). (b) H&E stain of a temporal artery affected by arteritis. Note the obliteration of the lumen by intimal inflammatory oedema/expansion. (c) H&E stain showing the adventitia (A) media (M), intima (I), and lumen (L) of a temporal artery affected by arteritis. Note the runs of inflammatory cells (small blue dots) in the media and adventitia. The lumen (L) is obliterated. (d) H&E stain of an inflamed temporal artery showing two multinucleate giant cells (left one indicated by arrow), that are present at the intima–media junction, accompanied by chronic inflammatory cells (lymphocytes, plasma cells, and histiocytes). (e) Elastin Van Gieson's stain (EVG) of a temporal artery affected by temporal arteritis. The asterisks indicate fragmentation and loss of the black elastin fibres.

Figure courtesy of Dr Hardeep Singh Mudhar, Consultant Ophthalmic Pathologist, Royal Hallamshire Hospital, Sheffield, UK.

Further reading

Chapter 9: Pathology. In: Forrester JV, Dick AD, McMenamin PG, Roberts F, Pearlman E. *The Eye: Basic Sciences in Practice* (4th Edition). Elsevier (2016).

45. C.

There are four main histological growth patterns for BCC: nodular, superficial, infiltrative, and basosquamous. The nodular and superficial growth patterns are associated with a low risk of recurrence, whereas the infiltrative (which encompasses micronodular, sclerosing, and infiltrating growth patterns) and basosquamous growth patterns are associated with a high risk of recurrence. Fig. 3.4 displays histopathological slides

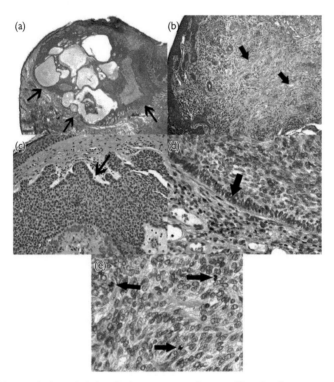

Figure 3.4 Histopathological slides displaying various forms of basal cell carcinoma (BCC). (a) Low-power haematoxylin and eosin (H&E) stain of an eyelid BCC of nodular-cystic type. The arrows outline the well-defined edge and the multiple cystic areas are seen in the tumour. (b) Low-power H&E stain of an eyelid BCC of infiltrative type, with arrows pointing to infiltrative tongues of basaloid cells present in a fibrotic surrounding stroma. (c) H&E stain of a BCC showing the retraction cleft that is often seen (arrow) between the tumour and the surrounding dermis. (d) H&E stain of BCC showing the palisade of cells (cells line up at right angles to the other tumour cells like a picket-fence) that is often seen along the perimeter of nodular and micronodular BCCs. (e) Higher power H&E stain of a BCC showing the basaloid tumour cells and mitotic figures (arrows).

Figure courtesy of Dr Hardeep Singh Mudhar, Consultant Ophthalmic Pathologist, Royal Hallamshire Hospital, Sheffield, UK.

Further reading

Chapter 9: Pathology. In: Forrester JV, Dick AD, McMenamin PG, Roberts F, Pearlman E. *The Eye: Basic Sciences in Practice* (4th Edition). Elsevier (2016).

Slater D, Barrett P. Royal College of Pathologists: dataset for histopathological reporting of primary cutaneous basal cell carcinoma. February 2019. https://www.rcpath.org/uploads/assets/53688094-791e-4aaa-82cec42c3cb65e35/Dataset-for-histopathological-reporting-of-primary-cutaneous-basal-cell-carcinoma.pdf Accessed 1 February 2021.

46. D.

The three steps of PCR are carried out in the following order: denaturation, annealing, and extension. Denaturation is followed by annealing of synthetic oligonucleotide primers, specifically designed to hybridise the target nucleic acid region. During a typical PCR analysis, 20–40 cycles are carried out, resulting in exponential amplification of the target region. Option D is true.

Further reading

Chapter 9: Pathology. In: Forrester JV, Dick AD, McMenamin PG, Roberts F, Pearlman E. *The Eye: Basic Sciences in Practice* (4th Edition). Elsevier (2016).

47. D.

A lymphocytic infiltrate typically appears around the long and short ciliary nerves in herpes zoster ophthalmicus.

Further reading

Chapter 9: Pathology. In: Forrester JV, Dick AD, McMenamin PG, Roberts F, Pearlman E. *The Eye: Basic Sciences in Practice* (4th Edition). Elsevier (2016).

48. D.

Due to age-related anteroposterior lens thickening and in small eyes, the anterior lens surface displaces the pupillary zone (not the peripheral zone) of the iris anteriorly.

Further reading

Chapter 9: Pathology. In: Forrester JV, Dick AD, McMenamin PG, Roberts F, Pearlman E. *The Eye: Basic Sciences in Practice* (4th Edition). Elsevier (2016).

49. C.

Macular dystrophy is inherited in an autosomal recessive manner, whereas lattice dystrophy, granular dystrophy, and Reis–Bücklers dystrophy are inherited in an autosomal dominant manner.

Further reading

Chapter 9: Pathology. In: Forrester JV, Dick AD, McMenamin PG, Roberts F, Pearlman E. *The Eye: Basic Sciences in Practice* (4th Edition). Elsevier (2016).

50. A.

Acute retinal necrosis usually occurs in immunocompetent individuals, whereas progressive outer retinal necrosis occurs in immunocompromised individuals.

Further reading

Chapter 9: Pathology. In: Forrester JV, Dick AD, McMenamin PG, Roberts F, Pearlman E. *The Eye: Basic Sciences in Practice* (4th Edition). Elsevier (2016).

51. D.

Regarding uveal melanoma, prognosis is worse in older patients, larger tumours, ciliary body location, epithelioid cell component, closed loop vascular pattern revealed on periodic acid–Schiff stain, monosomy 3 (or loss of heterozygosity of chromosome 3), and additional copies of chromosome 8q. Prognosis is more favourable in younger patients, smaller tumours, choroid location, tumours composed only of spindle cells, and aberrations/numerical gain of chromosome 6p.

Further reading

Chapter 9: Pathology. In: Forrester JV, Dick AD, McMenamin PG, Roberts F, Pearlman E. *The Eye: Basic Sciences in Practice* (4th Edition). Elsevier (2016).

Microbiology

52. C.

Pharyngoconjunctival fever is commonly caused by adenovirus serotypes 1, 2, 3, 5, 7, and 14. Epidemic keratoconjunctivitis is commonly caused by adenovirus serotypes 3, 7, 8, and 19.

Further reading

Chapter 8: Microbial infections of the eye. In: Forrester JV, Dick AD, McMenamin PG, Roberts F, Pearlman E. *The Eye: Basic Sciences in Practice* (4th Edition). Elsevier (2016).

53. C.

Pseudomonas aeruginosa is the most common cause of bacterial keratitis globally.

Further reading

Chapter 8: Microbial infections of the eye. In: Forrester JV, Dick AD, McMenamin PG, Roberts F, Pearlman E. *The Eye: Basic Sciences in Practice* (4th Edition). Elsevier (2016).

54. D.

If treatment is delayed, hyphae can penetrate into the anterior chamber, stimulating a neutrophil infiltrate (hypopyon) which limits further penetration to the posterior segment.

Further reading

Chapter 8: Microbial infections of the eye. In: Forrester JV, Dick AD, McMenamin PG, Roberts F, Pearlman E. *The Eye: Basic Sciences in Practice* (4th Edition). Elsevier (2016).

Immunology

55. C.

Tears contain lysozyme, which is effective against Gram-negative organisms and certain fungi. However, lysozyme is ineffective against Gram-positive organisms, such as *Staphylococcus aureus*.

Further reading

Chapter 7: Immunology. In: Forrester JV, Dick AD, McMenamin PG, Roberts F, Pearlman E. *The Eye: Basic Sciences in Practice* (4th Edition). Elsevier (2016).

56. D.

In Stevens–Johnson syndrome, the duration and degree of exposure to the causative drug affects the severity of the condition.

Further reading

Chapter 7: Immunology. In: Forrester JV, Dick AD, McMenamin PG, Roberts F, Pearlman E. *The Eye: Basic Sciences in Practice* (4th Edition). Elsevier (2016).

Pharmacology and genetics 3

Pharmacology

57. C.

A partial agonist is a ligand with both agonist and antagonist properties, thus it has a lower maximal effect than a pure agonist.

Further reading

Chapter 6: General and ocular pharmacology. In: Forrester JV, Dick AD, McMenamin PG, Roberts F, Pearlman E. *The Eye: Basic Sciences in Practice* (5th Edition). Elsevier (2021).

58. D.

Prostaglandin analogues (e.g. latanoprost) reduce intraocular pressure (IOP) mainly by increasing aqueous humour outflow via the uveoscleral (non-conventional) route. β-blockers (e.g. timolol) reduce aqueous production by up to 50%. Carbonic anhydrase inhibitors (e.g. acetazolamide) inhibit the activity of carbonic anhydrase in the ciliary body, thus reducing aqueous humour formation. Parasympathomimetics (e.g. pilocarpine) facilitate aqueous outflow by direct action on the scleral spur and ciliary body. α_2-adrenostimulants (e.g. brimonidine) facilitate aqueous outflow by stimulating receptors in the trabecular meshwork, increasing aqueous and intracellular cAMP.

Further reading

Chapter 6: General and ocular pharmacology. In: Forrester JV, Dick AD, McMenamin PG, Roberts F, Pearlman E. *The Eye: Basic Sciences in Practice* (5th Edition). Elsevier (2021).

59. A.

Systemic side effects of topical β-blockers include bradycardia, bronchospasm, syncope, and central nervous system depression. Facial flushing is a side effect of anti-muscarinic agents.

Further reading

Chapter 6: General and ocular pharmacology. In: Forrester JV, Dick AD, McMenamin PG, Roberts F, Pearlman E. *The Eye: Basic Sciences in Practice* (5th Edition). Elsevier (2021).

60. D.

Corticosteroids act on cytosolic receptors and block the transcription of cytokine genes. Ciclosporin inhibits calcineurin and nuclear factor of activated T cells (NFAT), thereby inhibiting interleukin-2 production. Azathioprine inhibits purine synthesis.

Further reading

Chapter 6: General and ocular pharmacology. In: Forrester JV, Dick AD, McMenamin PG, Roberts F, Pearlman E. *The Eye: Basic Sciences in Practice* (5th Edition). Elsevier (2021).

61. D.

α_1-receptors mediate excitatory responses (i.e. smooth muscle contraction) whereas α_2-receptors are inhibitory. β_1-receptors mediate excitatory responses of the heart (positive inotropic and chronotropic responses) whereas β_2-receptors are inhibitory (i.e. relaxation of the smooth muscle of blood vessels and bronchi). B_3-receptors are found in adipose tissue—they regulate lipolysis and thermogenesis.

Further reading

Chapter 6: General and ocular pharmacology. In: Forrester JV, Dick AD, McMenamin PG, Roberts F, Pearlman E. *The Eye: Basic Sciences in Practice* (5th Edition). Elsevier (2021).

62. C.

Ciproxifan is a histamine receptor antagonist that acts on H_3-receptors. Cetirizine, loratadine, and diphenhydramine act on H_1-receptors. Ranitidine and cimetidine act on H_2-receptors. Thioperamide acts on H_4-receptors.

Further reading

Chapter 6: General and ocular pharmacology. In: Forrester JV, Dick AD, McMenamin PG, Roberts F, Pearlman E. *The Eye: Basic Sciences in Practice* (5th Edition). Elsevier (2021).

Genetics

63. B.

The human haploid genome comprises 3×10^9 base pairs of **double**-stranded DNA (dsDNA). Most amino acids can be encoded by more than one codon, except methionine (ATG) and tryptophan (TGG). Exons are coding regions and introns are variable-length intervening regions of a gene.

Further reading

Chapter 3: Genetics. In: Forrester JV, Dick AD, McMenamin PG, Roberts F, Pearlman E. *The Eye: Basic Sciences in Practice* (5th Edition). Elsevier (2021).

64. D.

Inversions occur following two chromosomal breaks, where the segment is inverted **180°** between the two breaks.

Further reading

Chapter 3: Genetics. In: Forrester JV, Dick AD, McMenamin PG, Roberts F, Pearlman E. *The Eye: Basic Sciences in Practice* (5th Edition). Elsevier (2021).

65. B.

HLA-B27 is most strongly associated with ankylosing spondylitis and moderately associated with reactive arthritis. HLA-B51 is weakly associated with Behçet syndrome. HLA-B25 is weakly associated with acute anterior uveitis.

Further reading

Chapter 3: Genetics. In: Forrester JV, Dick AD, McMenamin PG, Roberts F, Pearlman E. *The Eye: Basic Sciences in Practice* (5th Edition). Elsevier (2021).

66. B.

GPR179 mutation is associated with congenital stationary night blindness.

Further reading

Chapter 3: Genetics. In: Forrester JV, Dick AD, McMenamin PG, Roberts F, Pearlman E. *The Eye: Basic Sciences in Practice* (5th Edition). Elsevier (2021).

67. C.

Liposomes can be employed as non-viral vectors for gene therapy. They are spherical lipid bilayer vesicles. Their **efficiency of transfer is low**, but they can accommodate DNA of any size.

Further reading

Chapter 3: Genetics. In: Forrester JV, Dick AD, McMenamin PG, Roberts F, Pearlman E. *The Eye: Basic Sciences in Practice* (5th Edition). Elsevier (2021).

68. B.

PITX2 mutation is associated with Axenfeld–Rieger syndrome. *OPA1* mutation is associated with dominant optic atrophy. *TIMP3* mutation is associated with Sorsby fundus dystrophy.

Further reading

Chapter 3: Genetics. In: Forrester JV, Dick AD, McMenamin PG, Roberts F, Pearlman E. *The Eye: Basic Sciences in Practice* (5th Edition). Elsevier (2021).

Investigations 3

69. D.

Glasses are used in the Titmus **and** TNO tests—the former requires polaroid glasses and the latter requires red–green glasses. The Lang test uses intrinsic cylinder lenses. The Frisby test uses intrinsic plate thickness.

Further reading

Denniston AKO, Wolffsohn J, Auld R, Murray PI. Chapter 1: Clinical skills. In: Denniston AKO, Murray PI. *Oxford Handbook of Ophthalmology*. Oxford University Press (2018).

70. B.

The Maddox rod test can be used to assess symptomatic phorias. The phoria can be quantified by neutralising prisms. A single Maddox rod (i.e. series of red cylinders) is positioned horizontally in front of the right eye fixing on a white spot. The line should pass through the spot if the patient has no horizontal phoria. If the line appears to the right of the white spot, the patient has right esophoria. If the line appears to the left of the white spot, the patient has right exophoria. The Maddox rod can be rotated vertically to identify vertical phorias.

Further reading

Denniston AKO, Wolffsohn J, Auld R, Murray PI. Chapter 1: Clinical Skills. In: Denniston AKO, Murray PI. *Oxford Handbook of Ophthalmology*. Oxford University Press (2018).

71. A.

Tilted disc syndrome arises due to congenital malformation of the optic nerve. Superior bitemporal field defects may be seen in approximately 20% of patients with tilted disc syndrome; importantly, these can cross the vertical meridian, whereas those in chiasmal lesions do not cross the vertical meridian.

Further reading

Mollan SP, Calcagni A, Keane PA. Chapter 2: Investigations and their interpretation. In: Denniston AKO, Murray PI. *Oxford Handbook of Ophthalmology*. Oxford University Press (2018).

72. C.

Anterior segment OCT is similar to posterior segment OCT, but the former uses longer-wavelength light (typically 1310 nanometres) than the latter (typically 800 nanometres). Fig. 3.5 and Fig. 3.6 display anterior segment OCT images of the cornea and iridocorneal angle, respectively.

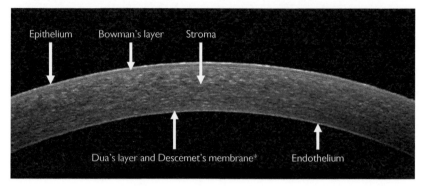

Figure 3.5 Anterior segment OCT image of the cornea, displaying normal anatomy. *It is difficult to distinguish the pre-Descemet's layer (Dua's layer) and Descemet's membrane on anterior segment OCT, as both have a similar refractive index, but easier to distinguish in cases of Descemet's membrane detachment where Dua's layer is involved (see Dua et al., 2020).

Image courtesy of Mr Dermot F. Roche, Vision Scientist, Great Ormond Street Hospital for Children, London.

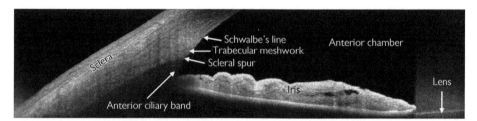

Figure 3.6 Anterior segment OCT image of the iridocorneal angle, displaying normal anatomy.

Image courtesy of Mr Dermot F. Roche, Vision Scientist, Great Ormond Street Hospital for Children, London.

Further reading

Dua HS, Faraj LA, Said DG, Gray T, Lowe J. Human corneal anatomy redefined: a novel pre-Descemet's layer (Dua's layer). *Ophthalmology*. 2013 Sep;*120*(9):1778–1785.

Dua HS, Sinha R, D'Souza S, et al. 'Descemet membrane detachment': a novel concept in diagnosis and classification. *Am J Ophthalmol*. 2020 Oct;*218*:84–98.

Mollan SP, Calcagni A, Keane PA. Chapter 2: Investigations and their interpretation. In: Denniston AKO, Murray PI. *Oxford Handbook of Ophthalmology*. Oxford University Press (2018).

73. A.

The phases of fundus fluorescein angiography are correctly ordered as follows: choroidal (pre-arterial), arterial, capillary, venous, and late.

Further reading

Mollan SP, Calcagni A, Keane PA. Chapter 2: Investigations and their interpretation. In: Denniston AKO, Murray PI. *Oxford Handbook of Ophthalmology*. Oxford University Press (2018).

74. C.

In ICG angiography, **leakage of dye** is commonly caused by choroidal neovascularisation, **abnormal blood vessels** are commonly caused by choroidal haemangioma, and **window defect** is commonly caused by retinal pigment epithelium defect.

Further reading

Mollan SP, Calcagni A, Keane PA. Chapter 2: Investigations and their interpretation. In: Denniston AKO, Murray PI. *Oxford Handbook of Ophthalmology*. Oxford University Press (2018).

75. B.

Fig. 1.6 (p. xxx) displays the layers of the retina on OCT. The correct order of the layers of the retina, from inner (closest to the vitreous) to outer (closest to the choroid), is as follows: **I**nner limiting membrane, **N**erve fibre layer, **G**anglion cell layer, **I**nner plexiform layer, **I**nner nuclear layer, **O**uter plexiform layer, **O**uter nuclear layer, **E**xternal limiting membrane, **P**hotoreceptor layer, **R**etinal pigment epithelium. A helpful mnemonic to remember this is as follows: **I**n **N**ew **G**eneration, **I**t **I**sn't **O**nly **O**phthalmologists **E**xamining **P**atients' **R**etinae.

Further reading

Mollan SP, Calcagni A, Keane PA. Chapter 2: Investigations and their interpretation. In: Denniston AKO, Murray PI. *Oxford Handbook of Ophthalmology*. Oxford University Press (2018).

76. D.

A higher-frequency ultrasonic transducer (8–10 MHz) is used in ocular ultrasonography (US), as compared to orbital US (3–5 MHz). Lower frequency permits enhanced depth penetration in orbital US, which can be used to assess orbital tumours and orbital disease such as thyroid eye disease. Ocular US (A-scan) is useful for measuring axial length, anterior chamber depth, and intraocular mass thickness. Ocular US (B-scan) is useful for detecting posterior segment pathology where media opacity (e.g. dense cataract, vitreous haemorrhage) obstructs fundal view, characterising intraocular masses, localising intraocular foreign bodies, and diagnosing calcified optic disc drusen.

Further reading

Mollan SP, Calcagni A, Keane PA. Chapter 2: Investigations and their interpretation. In: Denniston AKO, Murray PI. *Oxford Handbook of Ophthalmology*. Oxford University Press (2018).

77. B.

UBM uses a higher-frequency transducer (35–50 MHz) than standard ocular ultrasonography (8–10 MHz). UBM achieves higher-resolution imaging, typically achieving axial resolution of 30 micrometres and transverse resolution of 60 micrometres. However, depth penetration is less, making UBM suitable for anterior segment imaging.

Further reading

Mollan SP, Calcagni A, Keane PA. Chapter 2: Investigations and their interpretation. In: Denniston AKO, Murray PI. *Oxford Handbook of Ophthalmology*. Oxford University Press (2018).

78. A.

The risk of chloroquine/hydroxychloroquine retinopathy is dose and duration dependent. Functional loss of the parafovea is best localised with the spatial array of the multifocal electroretinogram comparing ring arrays. The central response (Ring 1) represents the central 3° of the visual field, while the next concentric ring (Ring 2) represents 3–10° from fixation. An early sign of chloroquine/hydroxychloroquine toxicity is depression of the response amplitude in Ring 2 with relative preservation of the central response in Ring 1.

Further reading

O'Neill EK, Smith R. Visual electrophysiology in the assessment of toxicity and deficiency states affecting the visual system. *Eye (Lond)*. 2021 Sep;*35*(9):2344–2353.

79. C.

When performing the EOG, the patient intermittently follows targets moving left to right over a 30° horizontal plane. The difference between the two electrodes is measured, with the electrode closest to the cornea most positive.

Further reading

Constable PA, Bach M, Frishman LJ, et al. ISCEV Standard for clinical electro-oculography (2017 update). *Documenta Ophthalmologica. Advances in Ophthalmology*. 2017 Feb;*134*(1):1–9.

Miscellaneous 3

80. C.

Sensitivity is the proportion of diseased people who test positive. Specificity is the proportion of people with a negative test who are healthy. Positive predictive value (PPV) is the probability that people who test positive truly have the disease. Negative predictive value (NPV) is the probability that people who test negative are truly healthy.

Further reading

Denniston AKO, Moseley M, Murray PI. Chapter 26: Evidence-based ophthalmology. In: Denniston AKO and Murray PI. *Oxford Handbook of Ophthalmology*. Oxford University Press (2018).

81. D.

CONSORT = Consolidated Standards of Reporting Trials. PRISMA = Preferred Reporting Items for Systematic Reviews and Meta-Analyses. See the EQUATOR Network website for other reporting guidelines with full details. STROBE = Strengthening the Reporting of Observational Studies in Epidemiology. STARD = Standards for Reporting of Diagnostic accuracy studies.

Further reading

EQUATOR Network. Enhancing the Quality and Transparency of Health Research. Available at: https://www.equator-network.org Accessed October 2021.

82. C.

The **mean** value is the 'average' value, which can be calculated by adding all the data points then dividing by the number of data points. The **median** value is the 'middle' value, which can be found using the following method: (i) order the data points from smallest to largest; (ii) add 1 to the total number of data points then halve this number; (iii) if the result is a whole number, such as 3, then the median value is the 3rd number, whereas if the result is a decimal number, such as 5.5, then the median value lies halfway between the 5th and 6th number (i.e. the average of these two numbers). The **mode** is the most frequently occurring number. Following the median value calculation method in this example, (i) order the data points from smallest to largest: 7, 11, 14, 16, 17, 19, 22, 28, 33, 42; (ii) there are 10 data points—add 1 to this value then halve to give 5.5; (iii) the median value is therefore the mean of the 5th and 6th data point, 17 and 19 respectively. Sum the two values and halve to give 18.

Further reading

Bunce C, Young-Zvandasara T. Simplified Ophthalmic Statistics (SOS) Part 2: How to summarise your data and why it's a good idea to do so. *Eye News*. 2018;25(2):34–35. Available at: https://www.eyen ews.uk.com/education/trainees/post/sos-simplified-ophthalmic-statistics-part-2-how-to-summarise-your-data-and-why-it-s-a-good-idea-to-do-so Accessed October 2021.

83. C.

In a normally distributed dataset, approximately:

- 68% of values lie within one standard deviation of the mean
- 95% of values lie within two standard deviations of the mean
- 99.7% of values lie within three standard deviations of the mean.

Further reading

Denniston AKO, Moseley M, Murray PI. Chapter 26: Evidence-based ophthalmology. In: Denniston AKO and Murray PI. *Oxford Handbook of Ophthalmology*. Oxford University Press (2018).

84. D.

In a landmark 1968 publication for the World Health Organization, Wilson and Junger stated ten principles for a good screening test:

1. The condition should be an **important** health problem.
2. There should be an **accepted** treatment for patients with recognised disease.
3. Facilities for **diagnosis and treatment** should be available.
4. There should be a **recognisable** latent or early symptomatic phase.
5. There should be a **suitable test** or examination.
6. The test should be **acceptable** to the population.
7. The **natural history** of the condition, including development from latent to declared disease, should be adequately understood.
8. There should be an agreed **policy** on whom to treat as patients.
9. The cost of case-finding (including a diagnosis and treatment of patients diagnosed) should be **economically balanced** in relation to possible expenditure on medical care as a whole.
10. Case-finding should be a **continuous** process and not a 'once and for all' project.

Source: Wilson JMG, Jungner G. *The Principles and Practice of Screening for Disease*. Geneva, Switzerland: World Health Organization; 1968. (Public Health Papers no. 34.)

Further reading

World Health Organization. *Screening Programmes: A Short Guide. Increase effectiveness, Maximize Benefits and Minimize Harm*. Copenhagen: WHO Regional Office for Europe; 2020.

85. C.

Fig. 1.10 (see p. xxx) is a flowchart displaying common statistical tests and rules.

Further reading

Bunce C, Young-Zvandasara T. Simplified Ophthalmic Statistics (SOS) Part 3: Which statistical test should I use (if any)? *Eye News*. 2019;25(4):34–36. Available at: https://www.eyenews.uk.com/educat ion/trainees/post/sos-simplified-ophthalmic-statistics-part-3-which-statistical-test-should-i-use-if-any Accessed November 2021.

86. C.

Fig. 1.10 (see p. xxx) is a flowchart displaying common statistical tests and rules.

Further reading

Bunce C, Young-Zvandasara T. Simplified Ophthalmic Statistics (SOS) Part 3: Which statistical test should I use (if any)? *Eye News.* 2019;25(4):34–36. Available at: https://www.eyenews.uk.com/educat ion/trainees/post/sos-simplified-ophthalmic-statistics-part-3-which-statistical-test-should-i-use-if-any Accessed November 2021.

87. D.

Detection bias occurs due to systematic differences between groups in how outcomes are determined. Recency bias occurs due to the tendency to favour recent events over older events. Lead-time bias occurs when earlier diagnosis of a disease falsely makes it seem like affected patients are surviving longer. Publication bias is a type of reporting bias, occurring where the outcome of the study influences the decision whether or not to publish it.

Further reading

Denniston AKO, Moseley M, Murray PI. Chapter 26: Evidence-based ophthalmology. In: Denniston AKO and Murray PI. *Oxford Handbook of Ophthalmology.* Oxford University Press (2018).

88.

  I.   A.

  II. D.

  III. B.

Equations for diagnostic accuracy testing:

$$Sensitivity = \frac{TP}{TP + FN}$$

$$Specificity = \frac{TN}{TN + FP}$$

$$PPV = \frac{TP}{TP + FP}$$

$$NPV = \frac{TN}{TN + FN}$$

$$Positive\ likelihood\ ratio = \frac{sensitivity}{1 - specificity}$$

$$Negative\ likelihood\ ratio = \frac{1 - sensitivity}{specificity}$$

$$Accuracy = \frac{TP + TN}{TP + TN + FP + FN}$$

Further reading

Denniston AKO, Moseley M, Murray PI. Chapter 26: Evidence-based ophthalmology. In: Denniston AKO and Murray PI. *Oxford Handbook of Ophthalmology.* Oxford University Press (2018).

Optics 4

1. **With respect to the eye, which of the following represents the main source of image imperfection when the pupil is small?**
   A. Spherical aberration
   B. Diffraction
   C. Chromatic aberration
   D. Stiles–Crawford effect

2. **Regarding testing stereoacuity, which statement is MOST likely to be correct?**
   A. The *Frisby* test consists of three clear plastic plates of the same thickness.
   B. The *TNO* test covers a range of 480–60 seconds of arc.
   C. Each test plate of the *Frisby* test features four squares filled with random shapes, of which three feature 'hidden' circles to be identified by the patient.
   D. The *Lang* stereotest requires red–green spectacles.

3. **Which of the following represents the image formed by a concave mirror where the object lies inside the principal focus?**
   A. Image real, inverted, and diminished
   B. Image virtual, erect, and enlarged
   C. Image real, erect, and enlarged
   D. Image virtual, inverted, and diminished

4. **Regarding thin prisms used for ophthalmic purposes, a prism of 1 prism dioptre power produces what angle of apparent deviation?**
   A. ¼°
   B. ½°
   C. ¾°
   D. 1°

MCQs for FRCOphth Part 1. Sohaib R. Rufai, Oxford University Press. © Oxford University Press 2023.
DOI: 10.1093/oso/9780192843715.003.0004

5. **Which of the following is the spherical equivalent of the following toric lens prescription: +2.00 DS/−1.00 DC?**

    A. +1.00 DS
    B. +1.50 DS
    C. +3.00 DS
    D. −1.00 DS

6. **Regarding the duochrome test, which statement is LEAST likely to be correct?**

    A. A myopic patient sees black letters on a red background letters more distinctly than black letters on a green background.
    B. The duochrome test is particularly useful in avoiding overcorrection of myopic patients.
    C. An overcorrected myopic patient may be using accommodation for distance vision, leading to eye strain.
    D. Colour blindness invalidates the duochrome test.

7. **Regarding accommodation, which statement is LEAST likely to be correct?**

    A. The near point of distinct vision is the nearest point an object can be seen clearly when maximal accommodation is used.
    B. The far point of the emmetropic eye is at infinity.
    C. The range of accommodation is the distance between the near point and far point.
    D. The dioptric power of the accommodated eye is called its static refraction.

8. **Regarding the pinhole occluder, which statement is MOST likely to be correct?**

    A. The pinhole occluder available clinically allows a single ray of light to pass through it.
    B. Refractive errors within the range +6 dioptres to −6 dioptres are corrected to 6/6 with a pinhole occluder.
    C. In macular disease, visual acuity may be worsened using a pinhole occluder as compared to the unaided acuity.
    D. The pinhole occluder cannot differentiate between refractive error and neurological disease.

9. **Approximately what degree of axial myopia is required to render the eye emmetropic without spectacles following cataract extraction, in dioptres (D)?**

    A. −10 to −12 D
    B. −14 to −16 D
    C. −18 to −20 D
    D. −22 to −24 D

10. **Regarding contact lenses versus spectacles, which of the following is LEAST likely to be true?**
    A. Rigid contact lenses cannot cause a halo effect.
    B. Spectacles are more likely to cause oblique aberrations than contact lenses.
    C. Spectacle lenses centred for distance may induce a prismatic effect on convergence of the eyes for reading.
    D. The field of view is reduced in hypermetropic individuals wearing spectacles.

11. **Regarding the use of the convex lens as a magnifying loupe, which statement is MOST likely to be correct?**
    A. The standard ×8 loupe possesses a lens power of 16 dioptres.
    B. The object is situated between the second principal focus and the lens.
    C. Bar-shaped convex cylindrical lenses used as reading aids produce a horizontal magnification of the letters when placed on a line of printed text.
    D. The field of vision obtained by a hand or stand magnifier depends on the size of the lens aperture and the eye–lens distance.

12. **What level of magnification is approximately achieved by the indirect ophthalmoscope when using a +13-dioptre condensing lens?**
    A. ×3
    B. ×4
    C. ×5
    D. ×6

13. **Regarding keratometry, which statement is LEAST likely to be true?**
    A. The anterior corneal surface acts as a convex mirror.
    B. The refractive index of tears is approximately 1.336.
    C. The peripheral cornea is more spherical than the central cornea.
    D. Light entering the peripheral cornea is normally screened off by the iris in an undilated pupil.

14. **Regarding the compound microscope, which statement is MOST likely to be true?**
    A. The objective lens is convex and the eyepiece lens is concave.
    B. The object is placed just inside the anterior focal point.
    C. The resulting image is virtual, inverted, and magnified.
    D. The resulting image is formed behind the objective lens.

15. **Regarding pachymetry, which statement is MOST likely to be true?**

    A. The Purkinje–Sanson images III and IV are used by the pachymeter to measure anterior chamber depth.
    B. The Maurice and Giardine pachymeter achieves image doubling by splitting the observer's view.
    C. The Jaeger pachymeter possess two glass plates, of which the lower plate is fixed.
    D. In ultrasound pachymetry, the probe only provides a reading when the probe is perpendicular to the anterior corneal surface.

16. **What is the wavelength emitted by neodymium–yttrium aluminium garnet (Nd-YAG) laser, in nanometres (nm)?**

    A. 764 nm
    B. 864 nm
    C. 964 nm
    D. 1064 nm

Anatomy 4

17. **Which structure does NOT pass through the superior orbital fissure?**

    A. Superior ophthalmic vein
    B. Frontal nerve
    C. Nasociliary nerve
    D. Ophthalmic artery

18. **Regarding the eyelids, which statement is MOST likely to be true?**

    A. The plica semilunaris lies on the medial side of the caruncle.
    B. The eyelashes of the lower lid are typically longer than those of the upper lid.
    C. There are approximately 10–15 meibomian glands in each lid.
    D. The grey line marks the anterior boundary of the tarsal plate.

19. **Approximately what is the anteroposterior diameter of the emmetropic eyeball in millimetres (mm)?**

    A. 20 mm
    B. 22 mm
    C. 24 mm
    D. 26 mm

20. **Which rectus muscle has the longest tendon length?**

    A. Superior
    B. Inferior
    C. Lateral
    D. Medial

21. **Which of the following represents the order of the corneal layers, from anterior to posterior?**
    A. Epithelium, stroma, Bowman's layer, pre-Descemet's layer (Dua's layer), Descemet's membrane, endothelium
    B. Epithelium, Bowman's layer, stroma, pre-Descemet's layer (Dua's layer), Descemet's membrane, endothelium
    C. Epithelium, pre-Descemet's layer (Dua's layer), Descemet's membrane, stroma, Bowman's layer, endothelium
    D. Epithelium, stroma, pre-Descemet's layer (Dua's layer), Descemet's membrane, Bowman's layer, endothelium

22. **Regarding the cranial fossae, which statement is LEAST likely to be true?**
    A. The anterior cranial fossa is posteriorly bounded by the greater wing of sphenoid.
    B. The middle cranial fossa is posteriorly bounded by the superior borders of the petrous temporal bones.
    C. The middle cranial fossa possesses expanded lateral parts and a small median part.
    D. The posterior cranial fossa houses the brainstem and cerebellum.

23. **Regarding the ciliary muscle, which statement is LEAST likely to be true?**
    A. Postganglionic parasympathetic fibres from the short ciliary nerves innervate the ciliary muscle.
    B. Ciliary muscle contraction pulls the suspensory ligaments taught.
    C. The ciliary muscle is made up of smooth muscle fibres.
    D. The innermost ciliary muscle region is formed of circular fibres.

24. **Which of the following retinal layers is closest to the choroid?**
    A. External limiting membrane
    B. Photoreceptor layer
    C. Outer nuclear layer
    D. Nerve fibre layer

25. **Regarding the optic nerve, which statement is MOST likely to be true?**
    A. Posterior to the optic disc, the optic nerve fibres are myelinated by Schwann cells.
    B. The optic nerve is approximately 8 cm long.
    C. The optic nerve comprises approximately 1.2 million myelinated ganglion cell axons.
    D. Müller cells are present at the optic disc.

26. **Approximately what proportion of the eyeball is filled by the vitreous body?**
    A. 1/2
    B. 2/3
    C. 3/4
    D. 4/5

27. Which pair of eye movements occur at the transverse axis of Fick?

A. Abduction and adduction

B. Elevation and depression

C. Extorsion and intorsion

D. Excycloduction and incycloduction

28. Regarding the trochlear nerve, which statement is LEAST likely to be true?

A. It is the most slender cranial nerve.

B. It is the only cranial nerve that leaves the posterior surface of the brainstem.

C. Its nucleus is located in the midbrain at the level of the superior colliculus.

D. It runs forward through the lateral wall of the cavernous sinus.

29. Regarding the optic nerve, which statement is LEAST likely to be true?

A. The intraocular portion begins at the optic disc and terminates at the lamina cribrosa.

B. The optic nerve fibres are myelinated by oligodendrocytes as they traverse the lamina cribrosa.

C. 10% of the optic nerve axons originate from midget ganglion cells.

D. After leaving the optic canal, the optic nerve passes backward, upward, and medially to reach the optic chiasm.

30. Which of the extraocular muscles are NOT typically identifiable by the fifth gestational week?

A. Superior rectus

B. Superior oblique

C. Levator palpebrae superioris

D. Lateral rectus

Physiology 4

Physiology of the eye and vision

31. Which of the following represents the correct order of lacrimal drainage structures, from eye to nose?

A. Superior and inferior puncta, common canaliculus, superior and inferior canaliculi, nasolacrimal sac, plica lacrimalis, nasolacrimal duct

B. Superior and inferior canaliculi, superior and inferior puncta, common canaliculus, nasolacrimal duct, nasolacrimal sac, plica lacrimalis

C. Superior and inferior puncta, superior and inferior canaliculi, common canaliculus, nasolacrimal duct, plica lacrimalis, nasolacrimal sac

D. Superior and inferior puncta, superior and inferior canaliculi, common canaliculus, nasolacrimal sac, nasolacrimal duct, plica lacrimalis

32. Regarding the corneal epithelium, which statement is LEAST likely to be true?

A. It is composed of four to six cell layers.
B. It is approximately 50 micrometres in thickness.
C. It is devoid of melanocytes.
D. Its cell layers turn over every 2–3 days.

33. Which eponym is associated with a remnant of glial tissue on the optic disc, due to incomplete resorption of the fetal hyaloid artery?

A. Mittendorf
B. Cloquet
C. Wieger
D. Bergmeister

34. Regarding the absorption of light by the retinal pigment epithelium (RPE), which statement is MOST likely to be correct?

A. Energy from light focused onto the macula is absorbed by the melanin granula in the RPE, causing a reduction in the temperature of the RPE choroid complex.
B. The choriocapillaris has a lower relative blood perfusion than that of the kidney.
C. Venous blood from the choroid possesses an oxygen saturation of less than 40%.
D. Ascorbate and light energy are absorbed by the carotenoids lutein and zeaxanthin.

35. Which of the following does NOT occur during accommodation?

A. Lens diameter decreases.
B. The posterior lens surface moves posteriorly.
C. The thickness of the cortex increases.
D. The lens anterior surface curvature increases.

36. Regarding light energy, which of the following definitions is MOST likely to be correct?

A. 1 apostilb = 1 metre-candela
B. 1 lux = 1 lumen/m^2
C. 1 lambert = 1 lux at 1 cm distance for a perfectly diffusing light source on a surface at 1 cm
D. 1 troland = 1 candela/m^2 viewed through a pupil of 1 mm^2

General physiology

37. Regarding the motor unit, which statement is MOST likely to be true?

A. Large muscles that do not require fine control possess fewer muscle fibres per motor unit.
B. The soleus muscle possesses two to three muscle fibres per motor unit.
C. Muscles fibres in each motor unit overlap other motor units in microbundles of 80–100 fibres.
D. Interdigitation enables separate motor units to contract in support of one another.

38. Regarding cardiac muscle, which statement is LEAST likely to be true?

A. Atrial and ventricular muscles have a longer duration of contraction as compared to skeletal muscle.

B. The specialised excitatory and conductive fibres of the heart possess abundant contractile fibrils.

C. The Frank–Starling mechanism of the heart can be expressed by ventricular function curves.

D. The action potential of a ventricular muscle fibre averages 105 millivolts.

39. Regarding the regulation of ventilation, which statement is MOST likely to be true?

A. The ventral respiratory group is mainly responsible for inspiration.

B. The dorsal respiratory group is mainly responsible for expiration, rate, and depth of breathing.

C. Most of the dorsal respiratory group of neurons are situated within the nucleus of the tractus solitarius.

D. The pneumotaxic centre is located dorsally in the inferior portion of the pons.

40. Regarding the adrenal glands, which statement is MOST likely to be true?

A. The zona glomerulosa secretes cortisol and corticosterone.

B. The zona fasciculata secretes aldosterone.

C. The zona reticularis secretes dehydroepiandrosterone and androstenedione.

D. The medulla is functionally related to the parasympathetic nervous system.

Biochemistry

41. Regarding the endoplasmic reticulum, which statement is MOST likely to be correct?

A. The rough endoplasmic reticulum is the site of synthesis of triglycerides and steroids.

B. The rough endoplasmic reticulum is prominent in the retinal pigment epithelium and Meibomian gland cells.

C. The smooth endoplasmic reticulum is highly developed in secretory cells, including the lacrimal gland acinar cell.

D. The smooth endoplasmic reticulum plays a role in the trafficking and modification of lipids.

42. Regarding biochemical properties of the corneal epithelium, which statement is MOST likely to be true?

A. It is ten cell layers thick.

B. Basal epithelial cells are bound to the basement membrane of the anterior corneal stroma by tight junctions.

C. The corneal epithelium only absorbs long-wavelength light.

D. Corneal epithelial cells contain integrin receptors for basement membrane components, such as collagen, fibronectin, and laminin.

43. **Regarding the non-vascular functions of the choroid, which statement is LEAST likely to be true?**
    A. The choroid drains aqueous fluid via uveoscleral outflow, accounting for up to 10% of aqueous outflow in humans.
    B. The choroid controls scleral thickness by secreting growth factors.
    C. The choroid controls ocular temperature by dissipating heat from the eye.
    D. Intrinsic choroidal neurons may possess a role in controlling blood flow to the choroid via nitric oxide.

Pathology 4

General and ocular pathology

44. **Between which two retinal layers are hard drusen located in age-related macular degeneration?**
    A. Retinal pigment epithelium basement membrane and Bruch's membrane.
    B. Retinal pigment epithelium basement membrane and retinal pigment epithelium cell cytoplasm.
    C. Bruch's membrane and photoreceptor layer.
    D. Bruch's membrane and outer nuclear layer.

45. **Which of the following represents the MOST common protozoal parasite to infect the eye?**
    A. *Toxoplasma gondii*
    B. *Acanthamoeba* spp.
    C. *Toxocara canis*
    D. *Wuchereria* spp.

46. **Which of the following does NOT represent a risk factor for primary closed-angle glaucoma?**
    A. Short axial length
    B. Shallow anterior chamber depth
    C. Male sex
    D. Anteroposterior thickening of the lens

47. **Regarding anterior corneal dystrophies, which statement is LEAST likely to be true?**
    A. Electron microscopy reveals curly fibres within the superficial fibrous nodules in Thiel–Behnke dystrophy.
    B. Reis–Bücklers dystrophy is associated with fine reticular opacities in the superficial cornea in early adult life.
    C. Cogan's microcystic dystrophy is associated with the proliferation of cells and thickening of Bowman's layer.
    D. Meesmann's dystrophy is characterised by the formation of loops of basement membrane.

48. **Regarding Fuch's endothelial dystrophy, which statement is LEAST likely to be true?**
    A. It affects elderly patients.
    B. It affects males more than females.
    C. There is a reduction in the endothelial cell population.
    D. Descemet's membrane is thickened.

49. **Regarding progressive outer retinal necrosis, which statement is LEAST likely to be true?**
    A. It occurs in immunocompromised individuals.
    B. It is associated with vitritis.
    C. It can be caused by herpes zoster and herpes simplex viruses.
    D. Visual prognosis is generally poor.

50. **Regarding sebaceous gland carcinoma, which statement is LEAST likely to be true?**
    A. Prognosis is better than that of squamous cell carcinoma.
    B. It may be present in Muir–Torre syndrome.
    C. The nodular growth pattern features lobules of tumour cells with foamy or vacuolated cytoplasm.
    D. Diffuse tumours demonstrate Pagetoid spread.

51. **Regarding retinoblastoma, which statement is LEAST likely to be true?**
    A. The incidence is 1 in 20,000 live births.
    B. Its growth can be endophytic or exophytic.
    C. A Homer Wright rosette is a circle of cells limited internally by a continuous membrane.
    D. Fleurettes are commonly detected in irradiated tumours.

52. **Which human herpesvirus type causes Kaposi sarcoma?**
    A. 5
    B. 6
    C. 7
    D. 8

Microbiology

53. **Regarding *Pseudomonas aeruginosa* virulence factors, which statement is MOST likely to be true?**
    A. *Pseudomonas aeruginosa* produces exotoxins directly into host cells via its type II secretion system.
    B. Exoenzyme (Exo)-T and ExoS permit bacterial survival in neutrophils by inhibiting reactive oxygen species production.
    C. Cytotoxic strains express ExoS but not ExoU.
    D. ExoU inhibits cell migration and phagocytosis.

54. **Regarding trachoma, which statement is LEAST likely to be true?**
    A. It is caused by *Chlamydia trachomatis* serovars D–K.
    B. It represents the most prevalent microbial cause of blindness globally.
    C. Entropion is caused by the contraction of scar tissue.
    D. Trichiasis can cause corneal opacification.

Immunology

55. **Which of the following cells of the innate and acquired immune systems possess many mitochondria?**
    A. Mast cells
    B. Basophils
    C. Neutrophils
    D. Eosinophils

56. **Regarding the acquired immune system and the eye, which statement is LEAST likely to be true?**
    A. IgA is produced in the lacrimal gland by B cells.
    B. The corneal surface contains intraepithelial and stromal leucocytes, some of whom possess the characteristics of antigen-presenting cells.
    C. The lacrimal gland produces immunosuppressive cytokines.
    D. Eosinophil cationic protein levels in tears are reduced in vernal keratoconjunctivitis.

Pharmacology and genetics 4

Pharmacology

57. **Regarding pharmacodynamics, which statement is LEAST likely to be true?**
    A. Cyclic adenosine monophosphate is synthesised from adenosine triphosphate.
    B. Acetylcholine and glutamate are excitatory neurotransmitters.
    C. Adenyl cyclase acts as a secondary messenger.
    D. Intracellular calcium constitutes 10% of total calcium in the body.

58. **Regarding intraocular pressure (IOP)-lowering medication, which statement is MOST likely to be true?**
    A. β-blockers only reduce IOP in eyes with raised IOP.
    B. Prostaglandin analogues increase aqueous outflow via the conventional pathway.
    C. Parasympathomimetics act directly on the scleral spur and ciliary body.
    D. Apraclonidine is a carbonic anhydrase inhibitor.

59. **Which of the following is LEAST likely to represent a systemic side effect of carbonic anhydrase inhibitors?**

A. Calcium depletion

B. Dermatitis

C. Renal stones

D. Paraesthesia of the extremities

60. **What is the mode of action of tacrolimus?**

A. Inhibits purine synthesis

B. Inhibits interleukin-2

C. Inhibits dihydrofolate reductase

D. Blocks the *de novo* pathway of purine synthesis

61. **Which of the following represents a selective β_1-blocker?**

A. Timolol

B. Betaxolol

C. Carteolol

D. Levobunolol

62. **Which of the following eicosanoids causes vasodilation?**

A. Prostaglandin I_2

B. Leukotriene B_4

C. Leukotriene D_4

D. Thromboxane A_2

Genetics

63. **Regarding transcription, which statement is LEAST likely to be true?**

A. RNA polymerase binds to the promoter, signalling the unwinding of the DNA helix.

B. The exons are excised before the transcript leaves the nucleus.

C. mRNA serves as a template on cytoplasmic ribosomes for protein synthesis, upon leaving the nucleus.

D. Poly-A polymerase adds the poly-A tail following transcription.

64. **Which of the following represents a nonsense mutation?**

A. Single nucleotide change altering a critical splice junction.

B. Insertion of a repeated codon, thus interrupting the coding sequence.

C. Single nucleotide change leading to an amino acid substitution in the polypeptide chain.

D. Single nucleotide change resulting in a premature stop codon, causing a shortened polypeptide chain.

65. **Which of the following equations correctly represents the Hardy–Weinberg equilibrium, where _p_ = proportion of normal alleles and _q_ = proportion of abnormal alleles?**

A. $p + 2pq + q = 1$
B. $p^2 + 2pq + q = 1$
C. $p + 2pq^2 + q = 1$
D. $p^2 + 2pq + q^2 = 1$

66. **Regarding retinoblastoma, which statement is MOST likely to be correct?**

A. It is the second most common ocular malignancy of childhood.
B. Unilateral cases typically have a strong family history.
C. 40% of cases are inherited.
D. It affects males more than females.

67. **Regarding linkage analysis, which statement is LEAST likely to be true?**

A. Crossover between homologous chromosomes can occur at any point along the chromosome.
B. Gene loci are considered linked when their alleles do not demonstrate independent segregation during meiosis.
C. In family linkage studies, one locus is considered for the disease and the other for the trait.
D. During meiosis, the likelihood of genes being transmitted together is independent of their distance from one another.

68. **On a pedigree chart, what does a solid square box indicate?**

A. Carrier male
B. Carrier female
C. Affected male
D. Affected female

Investigations 4

69. Which structure is indicated by the grey arrow in the following image?

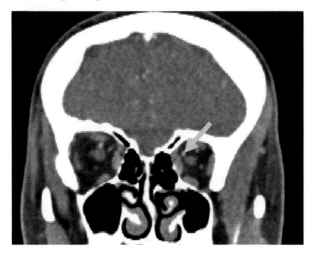

A. Left optic nerve
B. Left oculomotor nerve
C. Left ophthalmic artery
D. Left ophthalmic vein

70. Approximately how far does the temporal visual field extend?

A. 60°
B. 70°
C. 80°
D. 90°

71. Regarding global indices in Humphrey perimetry, which statement is LEAST likely to be true?

A. Mean deviation is a measure of overall field loss.
B. Short-term fluctuation indicates the consistency of responses.
C. Corrected pattern standard deviation corrects for short-term fluctuation.
D. A high pattern standard deviation is less indicative of glaucomatous field loss than mean deviation.

72. **Which of the following conditions is LEAST likely to be assessed by colour fundus photography?**
    A. Diabetic retinopathy screening
    B. Early diagnosis of peripheral retinal tears
    C. Monitoring patients taking chloroquine therapy
    D. Research studies for age-related macular degeneration

73. **In fundus fluorescein angiography, a window defect is MOST likely to be caused by which of the following conditions?**
    A. Drusen
    B. Tumour
    C. Macular hole
    D. Disciform scar

74. **Regarding optical reflectivity in optical coherence tomography (OCT), which of the following tissues are typically hyporeflective?**
    A. Inner plexiform layer
    B. Outer plexiform layer
    C. Inner nuclear layer
    D. Nerve fibre layer

75. **Regarding the optical coherence tomography (OCT) image of the macula below, what is the MOST likely diagnosis?**

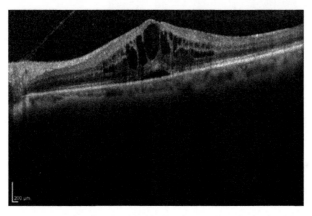

Reproduced with permission from Mollan SP, Calcagni A, Keane PA. Chapter 2: Investigations and their interpretation, Fig. 2.10, pg. 80. In: Denniston, AKO and Murray, PI (Eds) *Oxford Handbook of Ophthalmology*, 4th edition. 2018. Oxford, UK: Oxford University Press. Available at: https://global.oup.com/academic/.

    A. Macular hole
    B. Cystoid macular oedema
    C. Soft drusen
    D. Geographic atrophy

76. Regarding the principles of ocular ultrasonography, which statement is LEAST likely to be true?

A. When electrical voltage is applied across piezoelectric material, it expands or contracts at high frequency.

B. When sound waves are applied across piezoelectric material, it produces an electrical current.

C. The gain control can adjust the amount of ultrasonic energy emitted from the probe.

D. Ocular ultrasound delivers a lower axial resolution than optical coherence tomography.

77. Regarding the ocular ultrasound image (B-scan and vector A-scan) below, what is the MOST likely diagnosis?

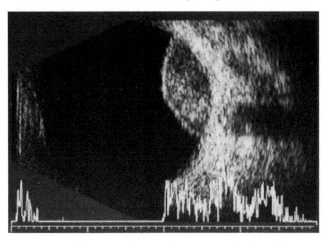

Investigations and their interpretation, Fig. 2.15, pg. 88. In: Denniston, AKO and Murray, PI (Eds) *Oxford Handbook of Ophthalmology*, 4th edition. 2018. Oxford, UK: Oxford University Press. Available at: https://global.oup.com/academic/.

A. Optic disc drusen

B. Posterior scleritis

C. Intraocular foreign body

D. Choroidal melanoma

78. Regarding the full-field electroretinogram (ERG), which statement is LEAST likely to be true?

A. It records mass retinal electrical activity upon stimulation by a flash of light.

B. Electrodes must be in contact with the cornea or nearby bulbar conjunctiva.

C. Dark adaptation takes 20 minutes.

D. The maximal ERG obtained after dark adaptation using a bright white flash is a pure rod response.

79. **Regarding the full-field electroretinogram, which of the following conditions is LEAST likely to cause reduced a- and b-waves?**
    A. Ophthalmic artery occlusion
    B. X-linked retinoschisis
    C. Metallosis
    D. Rod-cone dystrophy

Miscellaneous 4

80. **Which of the following equations is used to calculate number needed to treat?**
    A. 1/(Experimental event rate – Control event rate)
    B. 1/(Control event rate – Experimental event rate)
    C. Experimental event rate – Control event rate
    D. Control event rate – Experimental event rate

81. **On a Forest plot, what does the dashed vertical line represent?**
    A. Confidence intervals
    B. Line of no effect
    C. Overall meta-analysed measure of effect
    D. Study power

82. **What is denoted by the grey arrow on the following box and whisker plot?**

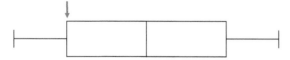

    A. Lowest value
    B. First quartile
    C. Third quartile
    D. Highest value

83. **What is the definition of severe distance visual impairment measured binocularly according to the International Classification of Diseases, 11th revision (ICD-11)?**

   A. Visual acuity worse than 6/12 to 6/18
   B. Visual acuity worse than 6/18 to 6/60
   C. Visual acuity worse than 6/60 to 3/60
   D. Visual acuity worse than 3/60

84. **According to the World Health Organization, approximately how many people worldwide have near or distance visual impairment?**

   A. 0.7 billion
   B. 1.2 billion
   C. 1.7 billion
   D. 2.2 billion

85. **What is the MOST appropriate statistical test to use for two groups where the outcome measure is continuous and the data are non-parametric and paired?**

   A. Wilcoxon signed rank test
   B. Kruskal–Wallis test
   C. Mann–Whitney U test
   D. Analysis of variance

86. **Regarding McNemar's test, which statement is MOST likely to be correct?**

   A. It should be used when the outcome measure is categorical and the data are paired.
   B. It should be used when the outcome measure is categorical and the data are unpaired.
   C. It should be used when the outcome measure is continuous and the data are non-parametric and paired.
   D. It should be used when the outcome measure is continuous and the data are non-parametric and unpaired.

87. **Which of the following options is MOST likely to cause attrition bias?**

   A. Unequal loss of participants from different arms of a trial.
   B. Failure to achieve proper randomisation during participant selection.
   C. The tendency to search for or favour information that confirms prior beliefs.
   D. Differences in the accuracy or completeness of recollections by participants regarding past events.

88. Regarding diagnostic accuracy testing:

I. Which of the following equations is used to calculate negative predictive value (NPV), where T = true, F = false, P = positives, and N = negatives?

A. $\dfrac{TP}{TP + FN}$

B. $\dfrac{TP}{TP + FP}$

C. $\dfrac{TN}{TN + FN}$

D. $\dfrac{TN}{TN + FP}$

II. Which of the following represents the correct formula for positive likelihood ratio?

A. $\dfrac{sensitivity}{1 - specificity}$

B. $\dfrac{1 - sensitivity}{1 - specificity}$

C. $\dfrac{1 - sensitivity}{specificity}$

D. $\dfrac{sensitivity}{specificity}$

III. Which of the following represents the correct formula for negative likelihood ratio?

A. $\dfrac{sensitivity}{specificity}$

B. $\dfrac{1 - sensitivity}{specificity}$

C. $\dfrac{sensitivity}{1 - specificity}$

D. $\dfrac{1 - sensitivity}{1 - specificity}$

Optics 4

1. B.

When the pupil is small, diffraction represents the main source of image imperfection. The Stiles–Crawford effect refers to the directional sensitivity of cone photoreceptors.

Further reading

Chapter 1: Properties of light and visual function. In: Elkington AR, Frank HJ, Greaney MJ. *Clinical Optics*. Blackwell Science (1999).

Chapter 8: Aberrations of optical systems including the eye. In: Elkington AR, Frank HJ, Greaney MJ. *Clinical Optics*. Blackwell Science (1999).

2. B.

The Frisby test consists of three clear plastic plates of different thicknesses. Each Frisby test plate features four squares, of which only **one** features a 'hidden' circle. The TNO test requires red–green spectacles.

Further reading

Chapter 1: Properties of light and visual function. In: Elkington AR, Frank HJ, Greaney MJ. *Clinical Optics*. Blackwell Science (1999).

3. B.

The image formed by the concave mirror where the object lies inside the principal focus is virtual, erect, and enlarged. Fig. 1.1 (see p. xxx) displays three ray diagrams for images formed by a concave mirror, depending on the position of the object. Fig. 1.2 (see p. xxx) displays a ray diagram for the image formed by a convex mirror.

Further reading

Chapter 2: Reflection of light. In: Elkington AR, Frank HJ, Greaney MJ. *Clinical Optics*. Blackwell Science (1999).

4. B.

Hence, 1 prism dioptre = ½°.

Further reading

Chapter 4: Prisms. In: Elkington AR, Frank HJ, Greaney MJ. *Clinical Optics*. Blackwell Science (1999).

5. B.

In a toric lens prescription, the spherical equivalent is the spherical power plus half the cylindrical power. Take care to handle the positive/negative signs correctly.

Further reading

Chapter 6: Astigmatic lenses. In: Elkington AR, Frank HJ. Greaney MJ. *Clinical Optics*. Blackwell Science (1999).

6. D.

Colour blindness does not invalidate the test—they can simply be asked whether the upper (red) or lower (green) rank of circles appears clearer (or letters, in older charts). The test makes use of the different wavelength foci of red and green light and the position of the image with respect to the retina.

Further reading

Chapter 8: Aberrations of optical systems including the eye. In: Elkington AR, Frank HJ, Greaney MJ. *Clinical Optics*. Blackwell Science (1999).

7. D.

The dioptric power of the resting eye is called its static refraction, whereas that of the accommodated eye is called its dynamic refraction. Other options are true.

Further reading

Chapter 9: Refraction by the eye. In: Elkington AR, Frank HJ, Greaney MJ. *Clinical Optics*. Blackwell Science (1999).

8. C.

The pinhole occluder available clinically allows a narrow pencil of light to pass through, rather than a single ray. Therefore, in high degrees of ametropia, the retinal image is too diffuse even when using the pinhole occluder to achieve 6/6 vision if the refractive error falls outside the range +4 dioptres to −4 dioptres. The pinhole occluder offers a simple and useful method to assess whether reduced visual acuity is due to refractive error as opposed to ocular pathology, including media opacities, or neurological disease.

Further reading

Chapter 10: Optics of ametropia. In: Elkington AR, Frank HJ, Greaney MJ. *Clinical Optics*. Blackwell Science (1999).

9. C.

If the degree of axial myopia is approximately −18 to −20 D, i.e. equal and opposite to the effective power of the extracted lens, then the eye is rendered emmetropic following cataract surgery.

Further reading

Chapter 10: Optics of ametropia. In: Elkington AR, Frank HJ, Greaney MJ. *Clinical Optics*. Blackwell Science (1999).

10. A.

Rigid contact lenses may cause a halo effect if the pupil is dilated, due to refraction of the peripheral lens or adjacent tear film.

Further reading

Chapter 12: Contact lenses. In: Elkington AR, Frank HJ, Greaney MJ. *Clinical Optics*. Blackwell Science (1999).

11. D.

The standard ×8 loupe possesses a lens power of 32 dioptres. The object is situated between the first principal focus and the lens. Bar-shaped convex cylindrical lenses used as reading aids produce a vertical magnification of the letters when placed on a line of printed text.

Further reading

Chapter 13: Optics of low vision aids. In: Elkington AR, Frank HJ, Greaney MJ. *Clinical Optics.* Blackwell Science (1999).

12. C.

In indirect ophthalmoscopy, the +13 D condensing lens approximately achieves ×5 magnification, while the +20 D condensing lens approximately achieves ×3 magnification.

Further reading

Chapter 14: Instruments. In: Elkington AR, Frank HJ, Greaney MJ. *Clinical Optics.* Blackwell Science (1999).

13. C.

The peripheral cornea is flatter than the central cornea. The central cornea, approximately 4 mm in diameter, is utilised for vision.

Further reading

Chapter 14: Instruments. In: Elkington AR, Frank HJ, Greaney MJ. *Clinical Optics.* Blackwell Science (1999).

14. D.

Both the objective lens and eyepiece lens are convex (option A is true for the Galilean telescope). The object is placed just outside the anterior focal point. The resulting image is real, inverted, and magnified.

Further reading

Chapter 14: Instruments. In: Elkington AR, Frank HJ, Greaney MJ. *Clinical Optics.* Blackwell Science (1999).

15. C.

The Purkinje–Sanson images II (posterior corneal surface) and III (anterior lens surface) are used by the pachymeter to measure anterior chamber depth. The Jaeger pachymeter achieves image doubling by splitting the observer's view, whereas the Maurice and Giardine pachymeter splits the incident light beam. In ultrasound pachymetry, the probe only provides a reading when the probe is perpendicular to the posterior corneal surface.

Further reading

Chapter 14: Instruments. In: Elkington AR, Frank HJ, Greaney MJ. *Clinical Optics.* Blackwell Science (1999).

16. D.

The Nd-YAG laser is commonly used to perform posterior capsulotomy and peripheral iridotomy. It emits 1064 nm infrared radiation.

Further reading

Chapter 15: Lasers. In: Elkington AR, Frank HJ, Greaney MJ. *Clinical Optics.* Blackwell Science (1999).

Anatomy 4

17. D.

The ophthalmic artery and optic nerve pass through the optic canal. The structures passing through the superior orbital fissure are as follows: lacrimal nerve, frontal nerve, trochlear nerve, superior ophthalmic vein, superior division of oculomotor nerve, nasociliary nerve, inferior division of oculomotor nerve, abducent nerve, and inferior ophthalmic vein.

Further reading

Chapter 1: Anatomy of the eye and orbit. In: Forrester JV, Dick AD, McMenamin PG, Roberts F, Pearlman E. *The Eye: Basic Sciences in Practice* (4th Edition). Elsevier (2016).

Chapter 3: The orbital cavity. In: Snell RS, Lemp MA. *Clinical Anatomy of the Eye* (2nd Edition). John Wiley and Sons (1998).

18. D.

The plica semilunaris lies on the lateral side of the caruncle. The eyelashes of the upper lid are typically longer and more numerous. There are approximately 30 meibomian glands in the upper lids and slightly fewer on the lower lids.

Further reading

Chapter 1: Anatomy of the eye and orbit. In: Forrester JV, Dick AD, McMenamin PG, Roberts F, Pearlman E. *The Eye: Basic Sciences in Practice* (4th Edition). Elsevier (2016).

Chapter 5: The ocular appendages. In: Snell RS, Lemp MA. *Clinical Anatomy of the Eye* (2nd Edition). John Wiley and Sons (1998).

19. C.

The approximate anteroposterior diameter of the emmetropic eyeball is 24 mm, while the vertical diameter is approximately 23 mm and the horizontal diameter approximately 23.5 mm.

Further reading

Chapter 6: The eyeball. In: Snell RS, Lemp MA. *Clinical Anatomy of the Eye* (2nd Edition). John Wiley and Sons (1998).

20. C.

The approximate rectus muscle tendon lengths are as follows, from longest to shortest: lateral, 8.8 mm; superior: 5.8 mm; inferior: 5.5 mm; medial: 3.7 mm. Please note that different textbooks quote slightly different measurements.

Further reading

Chapter 6: The eyeball. In: Snell RS, Lemp MA. *Clinical Anatomy of the Eye* (2nd Edition). John Wiley and Sons (1998).

21. B.

Dua's layer was published in *Ophthalmology* in 2013. See Fig. 3.5 (p. xxx) for anterior segment optical coherence tomography of the cornea.

Further reading

Dua HS, Faraj LA, Said DG, Gray T, Lowe J. Human corneal anatomy redefined: a novel pre-Descemet's layer (Dua's layer). *Ophthalmology*. 2013 Sep;120(9):1778–1785.

22. A.

The anterior cranial fossa is posteriorly bounded anteriorly by the frontal bone and posteriorly by the sharp lesser wing of sphenoid.

Further reading

Chapter 1: An overview of the anatomy of the skull. In: Snell RS, Lemp MA. *Clinical Anatomy of the Eye* (2nd Edition). John Wiley and Sons (1998)

23. B.

Ciliary muscle contraction pulls the ciliary body anteriorly, which relaxes the suspensory ligaments and causes the lens to become more convex, thus increasing its refractive power in accommodation. From externally to internally, its muscle fibres can be categorised as longitudinal (or meridonial), radial (or oblique), and circular.

Further reading

Chapter 6: The eyeball. In: Snell RS, Lemp MA. *Clinical Anatomy of the Eye* (2nd Edition). John Wiley and Sons (1998).

24. B.

Fig. 1.6 (see p. xxx) displays the layers of the retina as seen on optical coherence tomography (OCT). The correct order of the layers of the retina, from inner (closest to the vitreous) to outer (closest to the choroid), is as follows: **I**nternal limiting membrane, **N**erve fibre layer, **G**anglion cell layer, **I**nner plexiform layer, **I**nner nuclear layer, **O**uter plexiform layer, **O**uter nuclear layer, **E**xternal limiting membrane, **E**llipsoid zone, **R**etinal pigment epithelium. A helpful mnemonic to remember this is as follows: **I**n **N**ew **G**eneration, **I**t **I**sn't **O**nly **O**phthalmologists **E**xamining **E**very **R**etina.

Further reading

Chapter 6: The eyeball. In: Snell RS, Lemp MA. *Clinical Anatomy of the Eye* (2nd Edition). John Wiley and Sons (1998).

25. C.

Posterior to the optic disc, the optic nerve fibres are myelinated by oligodendrocytes, not Schwann cells, because the optic nerve is akin to a central nervous system tract. The optic nerve is approximately 4 cm long. Unlike the surrounding retina, there are no Müller cells present at the optic disc. Müller cells are the principal glial cells of the retina.

Further reading

Chapter 6: The eyeball. In: Snell RS, Lemp MA. *Clinical Anatomy of the Eye* (2nd Edition). John Wiley and Sons (1998).

26. D.

The vitreous body fills the eyeball between the retina and lens, occupying approximately four-fifths of the eyeball.

Further reading

Chapter 6: The eyeball. In: Snell RS, Lemp MA. *Clinical Anatomy of the Eye* (2nd Edition). John Wiley and Sons (1998).

27. B.

The three axes of Fick are as follows: (i) vertical; (ii) transverse; and (iii) sagittal. The respective eye movements about these three axes are as follows: (i) abduction and adduction; (ii) elevation and depression; and (iii) extorsion and intorsion. Excycloduction and incycloduction are alternative terms for extorsion and intorsion respectively.

Further reading

Chapter 8: Movements of the eyeball and the extraocular muscles. In: Snell RS, Lemp MA. *Clinical Anatomy of the Eye* (2nd Edition). John Wiley and Sons (1998).

28. C.

Its nucleus is located in the midbrain at the level of the inferior colliculus.

Further reading

Chapter 10: Cranial nerves—part 1: the nerves directly associated with the eye and orbit. In: Snell RS, Lemp MA. *Clinical Anatomy of the Eye* (2nd Edition). John Wiley and Sons (1998).

29. C.

Approximately 90% of the optic nerve axons originate from midget ganglion cells associated with cones, hence they are of small diameter (1 micrometre), whereas 10% of axons are related to ganglion cells associated with rods from the peripheral retina, hence they are of larger diameter (2 to 10 micrometres).

Further reading

Chapter 13: The visual pathway. In: Snell RS, Lemp MA. *Clinical Anatomy of the Eye* (2nd Edition). John Wiley and Sons (1998).

30. B.

The extraocular muscles are identifiable in roughly the following order: lateral rectus, superior rectus, levator palpebrae superioris at week 5; superior oblique and medial rectus at week 6; followed by interior oblique and inferior rectus.

Further reading

Chapter 1: Anatomy of the eye and orbit. In: Forrester JV, Dick AD, McMenamin PG, Roberts F, Pearlman E. *The Eye: Basic Sciences in Practice* (4th Edition). Elsevier (2016).

Physiology 4

Physiology of the eye and vision

31. D.

The correct order of lacrimal drainage structures, from eye to nose, are as follows: superior and inferior puncta, superior and inferior canaliculi, common canaliculus, nasolacrimal sac, nasolacrimal duct, plica lacrimalis.

Further reading

Chapter 5: The ocular appendages. In: Snell RS, Lemp MA. *Clinical Anatomy of the Eye* (2nd Edition). John Wiley and Sons (1998).

Dartt DA. Chapter 15: Formation and function of the tear film. In: Levin LA, Nilsson SFE, Ver Hoeve J, et al. *Adler's Physiology of the Eye* (11th Edition). Elsevier (2011).

32. D.

The cell layers of the corneal epithelium turn over approximately every 7–10 days. To maintain a smooth and uniform corneal epithelial surface, there is a fine balance of shedding and proliferation.

Further reading

Dawson DG, Ubels JL, Edelhauser HF. Chapter 4: Cornea and sclera. In: Levin LA, Nilsson SFE, Ver Hoeve J, et al. *Adler's Physiology of the Eye* (11th Edition). Elsevier (2011).

33. D.

Bergmeister's papilla is a small remnant of glial tissue on the optic disc, while Mittendorf's dot is a small, circular opacity found on the posterior lens capsule—both represent remnants of the fetal hyaloid artery. Cloquet's canal serves as a perivascular sheath for the fetal hyaloid artery, formed by an invagination of the hyaloid membrane. Wieger's ligament represents the attachment of the vitreous to the lens.

Further reading

Lund-Anderson H, Sander B. Chapter 6: The vitreous. In: Levin LA, Nilsson SFE, Ver Hoeve J, et al. *Adler's Physiology of the Eye* (11th Edition). Elsevier (2011).

34. D.

Energy from light focused onto the macula is absorbed by the melanin granula in the RPE, causing an increase in the temperature of the RPE choroid complex. The choriocapillaris has a **higher** relative blood perfusion than that of the kidney. Venous blood from the choroid possesses an oxygen saturation of **over 90%**.

Further reading

Strauss O, Helbig H. Chapter 13: The function of the retinal pigment epithelium. In: Levin LA, Nilsson SFE, Ver Hoeve J, et al. *Adler's Physiology of the Eye* (11th Edition). Elsevier (2011).

35. C.

During accommodation, the thickness of the nucleus increases but the thickness of the cortex does not change.

Further reading

Glasser A. Chapter 3: Accommodation. In: Levin LA, Nilsson SFE, Ver Hoeve J, et al. *Adler's Physiology of the Eye* (11th Edition). Elsevier (2011).

36. D.

1 apostilb = 1 lumen/m². 1 lux = 1 metre-candela. 1 lambert = 1 candela at 1 cm distance for a perfectly diffusing light source on a surface at 1 cm. Please note that the term 'apostilb' is now obsolete.

Further reading

Chapter 1: Properties of light and visual function. In: Elkington AR, Frank HJ, Greaney MJ. *Clinical Optics*. Blackwell Science (1999).

Chapter 5: Physiology of vision and the visual system. In: Forrester JV, Dick AD, McMenamin PG, Roberts F, Pearlman E. *The Eye: Basic Sciences in Practice* (4th Edition). Elsevier (2016).

General physiology

37. D.

A motor unit comprises all the muscle fibres innervated by a single nerve fibre. Larger muscles that do not require fine control (e.g. the soleus muscle) possess several hundred muscle fibres per motor unit, whereas smaller muscles that require fine control (e.g. some of the laryngeal muscles) possess only two or three muscles per motor unit. Muscle fibres in each motor unit overlap other motor units in microbundles of 3–15 fibres. On average, there are approximately 80–100 muscle fibres per motor unit throughout the human body.

Further reading

Chapter 6: Contraction of skeletal muscle. In: Hall JE. *Guyton and Hall Textbook of Medical Physiology* (13th Edition). Elsevier (2016).

38. B.

The specialised excitatory and conductive fibres of the heart possess few contractile fibrils and hence contract weakly. They provide an excitatory system that governs the rhythmical beating of the heart. The Frank–Starling mechanism of the heart states that the more the cardiac muscle is stretched during filling, the greater the force of contraction and the greater the volume of blood pumped into the aorta.

Further reading

Chapter 9: Cardiac muscle; the heart as a pump and function of the heart valves. In: Hall JE. *Guyton and Hall Textbook of Medical Physiology* (13th Edition). Elsevier (2016).

39. C.

The dorsal respiratory group is mainly responsible for inspiration. The ventral respiratory group is mainly responsible for expiration. The pneumotaxic centre is located dorsally in the superior (not inferior) portion of the pons. The pneumotaxic centre governs the rate and depth of breathing.

Further reading

Chapter 42: Regulation of respiration. In: Hall JE. *Guyton and Hall Textbook of Medical Physiology* (13th Edition). Elsevier (2016).

40. C.

The zona glomerulosa secretes aldosterone. The zona fasciculata secretes cortisol and corticosterone, plus small quantities of adrenal androgens and oestrogens. The zona reticularis secretes dehydroepiandrosterone and androstenedione, plus small quantities of oestrogens and some glucocorticoids. The medulla is functionally related to the sympathetic nervous system and secretes adrenaline and noradrenaline.

Further reading

Chapter 78: Adrenocortical hormones. In: Hall JE. *Guyton and Hall Textbook of Medical Physiology* (13th Edition). Elsevier (2016).

Biochemistry

41. D.

The **smooth** endoplasmic reticulum is the site of synthesis of lipids, triglycerides, and steroids; it is prominent in the retinal pigment epithelium and meibomian gland cells. The **rough** endoplasmic reticulum is a ribosome-studded structure, highly developed in secretory cells, including the lacrimal gland acinar cell.

Further reading

Chapter 4: Biochemistry and cell biology. In: Forrester JV, Dick AD, McMenamin PG, Roberts F, Pearlman E. *The Eye: Basic Sciences in Practice* (5th Edition). Elsevier (2021).

42. D.

The corneal epithelium is **six** cell layers thick. Basal epithelial cells are bound to the basement membrane of the anterior corneal stroma by **hemidesmosomes**. The corneal epithelia layer performs most of the light-absorbing properties of the cornea, mainly for short-wavelength light, though it does transmit electromagnetic radiation on the visible spectrum.

Further reading

Chapter 4: Biochemistry and cell biology. In: Forrester JV, Dick AD, McMenamin PG, Roberts F, Pearlman E. *The Eye: Basic Sciences in Practice* (5th Edition). Elsevier (2021).

43. A.

The choroid drains aqueous fluid from the anterior segment via uveoscleral outflow, accounting for up to **40%** of aqueous outflow in humans.

Further reading

Chapter 4: Biochemistry and cell biology. In: Forrester JV, Dick AD, McMenamin PG, Roberts F, Pearlman E. *The Eye: Basic Sciences in Practice* (5th Edition). Elsevier (2021).

Pathology 4

General and ocular pathology

44. A.

In age-related macular degeneration, hard and soft drusen are located between the retinal pigment epithelium (RPE) basement membrane and Bruch's membrane, whereas basal linear deposit occurs between the RPE basement membrane and RPE cell cytoplasm.

Further reading

Chapter 9: Pathology. In: Forrester JV, Dick AD, McMenamin PG, Roberts F, Pearlman E. *The Eye: Basic Sciences in Practice* (4th Edition). Elsevier (2016).

45. A.

Toxoplasma gondii represents the most common protozoal parasite to infect the eye. Congenital infection can occur if a woman is first infected during pregnancy. The classical tetrad of clinical features are as follows: meningoencephalitis, hydrocephalus, intracranial calcification, and retinochoroiditis.

Further reading

Chapter 9: Pathology. In: Forrester JV, Dick AD, McMenamin PG, Roberts F, Pearlman E. *The Eye: Basic Sciences in Practice* (4th Edition). Elsevier (2016).

46. C.

Risk factors for primary closed-angle glaucoma include advancing age, female sex, family history of primary angle-closure glaucoma, hypermetropia, shallow anterior chamber depth, short axial length, and anteroposterior thickening of the lens. Patients of East Asian descent may be at risk of a less acute and sometimes painless form of chronic angle closure glaucoma.

Further reading

Chapter 9: Pathology. In: Forrester JV, Dick AD, McMenamin PG, Roberts F, Pearlman E. *The Eye: Basic Sciences in Practice* (4th Edition). Elsevier (2016).

47. C.

Cogan's microcystic dystrophy is associated with degeneration of cells with cyst formation, causing an unstable corneal epithelium.

Further reading

Chapter 9: Pathology. In: Forrester JV, Dick AD, McMenamin PG, Roberts F, Pearlman E. *The Eye: Basic Sciences in Practice* (4th Edition). Elsevier (2016).

48. B.

Fuch's endothelial dystrophy is a common corneal dystrophy that affects females more than males.

Further reading

Chapter 9: Pathology. In: Forrester JV, Dick AD, McMenamin PG, Roberts F, Pearlman E. *The Eye: Basic Sciences in Practice* (4th Edition). Elsevier (2016).

49. B.

Unlike acute retinal necrosis, progressive outer retinal necrosis is not associated with papillitis, retinal vasculitis, or papillitis.

Further reading

Chapter 9: Pathology. In: Forrester JV, Dick AD, McMenamin PG, Roberts F, Pearlman E. *The Eye: Basic Sciences in Practice* (4th Edition). Elsevier (2016).

50. A.

Often heralded as 'the great masquerader', sebaceous gland carcinoma can often be indistinguishable from basal cell carcinoma, squamous cell carcinoma (SCC), or can masquerade as benign conditions such as blepharoconjunctivitis or chalazion. Prognosis is poorer than most other eyelid cancers, including SCC, with a relatively high risk of recurrence. Prognosis is improved by early recognition and surgical treatment. Histological growth patterns may be nodular or diffuse and tumours may be well, moderately, or poorly differentiated.

Further reading

Chapter 9: Pathology. In: Forrester JV, Dick AD, McMenamin PG, Roberts F, Pearlman E. *The Eye: Basic Sciences in Practice* (4th Edition). Elsevier (2016).

51. C.

Retinoblastoma may demonstrate endophytic growth (into the vitreous) or exophytic growth (into the subretinal space). Histologically, its differentiation may be seen in the form of Homer Wright rosettes, Flexner–Wintersteiner rosettes (described in option C), or fleurettes. Homer Wright rosettes are seen as a multilayered circle of nuclei surrounding eosinophilic fibrillate material, with no lumen or internal limiting membrane. Fleurettes are primitive photoreceptor bodies, arranged in a 'fleur de lys' shape.

Further reading

Chapter 9: Pathology. In: Forrester JV, Dick AD, McMenamin PG, Roberts F, Pearlman E. *The Eye: Basic Sciences in Practice* (4th Edition). Elsevier (2016).

52. D.

Kaposi sarcoma is a rare vascular tumour of endothelial cells, common in immunocompromised individuals, particularly those with AIDS. It is caused by human herpesvirus type 8.

Further reading

Chapter 9: Pathology. In: Forrester JV, Dick AD, McMenamin PG, Roberts F, Pearlman E. *The Eye: Basic Sciences in Practice* (4th Edition). Elsevier (2016).

Microbiology

53. B.

Pseudomonas aeruginosa produces exotoxins directly into host cells via its type III secretion system (T3SS). Cytotoxic strains express ExoU but not ExoS, while ExoS-expressing strains are invasive. ExoU is responsible for rapid cell lysis, while ExoS and ExoT have ADP-ribosyl transferase and GTPase-activating protein enzymatic activity, which inhibits cell migration and phagocytosis. This is achieved through blocking cytoskeleton activity.

Further reading

Chapter 8: Microbial infections of the eye. In: Forrester JV, Dick AD, McMenamin PG, Roberts F, Pearlman E. *The Eye: Basic Sciences in Practice* (4th Edition). Elsevier (2016).

54. A.

Trachoma is caused by *Chlamydia trachomatis* serovars A–C, whereas serovars D–K cause urogenital tract infections.

Further reading

Chapter 8: Microbial infections of the eye. In: Forrester JV, Dick AD, McMenamin PG, Roberts F, Pearlman E. *The Eye: Basic Sciences in Practice* (4th Edition). Elsevier (2016).

Immunology

55. B.

Basophils possess two to three nuclear lobes and feature many mitochondria and ribosomes, large coarse granules, and glycogen in abundance. By contrast, mast cells neutrophils, and eosinophils all possess few mitochondria.

Further reading

Chapter 7: Immunology. In: Forrester JV, Dick AD, McMenamin PG, Roberts F, Pearlman E. *The Eye: Basic Sciences in Practice* (4th Edition). Elsevier (2016).

56. D.

Eosinophil cationic protein levels in tears are significantly increased in both vernal and atopic keratoconjunctivitis.

Further reading

Chapter 7: Immunology. In: Forrester JV, Dick AD, McMenamin PG, Roberts F, Pearlman E. *The Eye: Basic Sciences in Practice* (4th Edition). Elsevier (2016).

Pharmacology and genetics 4

Pharmacology

57. D.

Intracellular calcium constitutes approximately 1% of total calcium in the body; hydroxyapatite in the bones and teeth constitutes approximately 99% of total body calcium.

Further reading

Chapter 6: General and ocular pharmacology. In: Forrester JV, Dick AD, McMenamin PG, Roberts F, Pearlman E. *The Eye: Basic Sciences in Practice* (5th Edition). Elsevier (2021).

58. C.

β-blockers reduce IOP even in **healthy** eyes by decreasing aqueous production by up to 50%. Prostaglandin analogues increase aqueous outflow via the **non-conventional** (uveoscleral) pathway. Apraclonidine is a **parasympathomimetic**.

Further reading

Chapter 6: General and ocular pharmacology. In: Forrester JV, Dick AD, McMenamin PG, Roberts F, Pearlman E. *The Eye: Basic Sciences in Practice* (5th Edition). Elsevier (2021).

59. A.

Carbonic anhydrase inhibitors can cause **potassium** depletion. Other systemic side effects include fatigue and acidosis.

Further reading

Chapter 6: General and ocular pharmacology. In: Forrester JV, Dick AD, McMenamin PG, Roberts F, Pearlman E. *The Eye: Basic Sciences in Practice* (5th Edition). Elsevier (2021).

60. B.

Tacrolimus inhibits interleukin-2. Azathioprine inhibits purine synthesis. Methotrexate (folic acid antagonist) inhibits dihydrofolate reductase and suppresses DNA synthesis. Mycophenolate (CellCept®) blocks the *de novo* pathway of purine synthesis (selective for lymphocytes).

Further reading

Chapter 6: General and ocular pharmacology. In: Forrester JV, Dick AD, McMenamin PG, Roberts F, Pearlman E. *The Eye: Basic Sciences in Practice* (5th Edition). Elsevier (2021).

61. B.

Betaxolol is a selective β_1-blocker. Timolol, carteolol, and levobunolol are non-selective β-blockers (i.e. β_1 and β_2).

Further reading

Chapter 6: General and ocular pharmacology. In: Forrester JV, Dick AD, McMenamin PG, Roberts F, Pearlman E. *The Eye: Basic Sciences in Practice* (5th Edition). Elsevier (2021).

62. A.

Prostaglandin I_2 causes vasodilation and reduces platelet adhesion. Prostaglandin F_{2a} causes bronchial smooth muscle contraction. Prostaglandin E_2 causes vasodilation, bronchodilation, uterine contraction, fever, macrophage activation, and release of pituitary hormones, adrenal cortex steroids, and insulin from the pancreas. Leukotriene B_4 causes aggregation of neutrophils, chemotaxis, and stimulation of phospholipase A_2. Leukotriene D_4 causes contraction of smooth muscle, vasoconstriction, and bronchoconstriction. Thromboxane A_2 causes vasoconstriction, bronchoconstriction, and platelet aggregation.

Further reading

Chapter 6: General and ocular pharmacology. In: Forrester JV, Dick AD, McMenamin PG, Roberts F, Pearlman E. *The Eye: Basic Sciences in Practice* (5th Edition). Elsevier (2021).

Genetics

63. B.

Before the transcript leaves the nucleus, the introns are excised while the exons are ligated together.

Further reading

Chapter 3: Genetics. In: Forrester JV, Dick AD, McMenamin PG, Roberts F, Pearlman E. *The Eye: Basic Sciences in Practice* (5th Edition). Elsevier (2021).

64. D.

A single nucleotide change altering a critical splice junction can cause a splice site mutation. Insertion of a repeated codon, thus interrupting the coding sequence, causes repeat expansions. A single nucleotide change leading to an amino acid substitution in the polypeptide chain causes a missense mutation.

Further reading

Chapter 3: Genetics. In: Forrester JV, Dick AD, McMenamin PG, Roberts F, Pearlman E. *The Eye: Basic Sciences in Practice* (5th Edition). Elsevier (2021).

65. D.

The Hardy–Weinberg equilibrium asserts that genetic variation of a population remains constant from one generation to the next, in the absence of disturbing factors such as mutation and selection.

Further reading

Chapter 3: Genetics. In: Forrester JV, Dick AD, McMenamin PG, Roberts F, Pearlman E. *The Eye: Basic Sciences in Practice* (5th Edition). Elsevier (2021).

66. C.

Retinoblastoma is a tumour of primitive photoreceptor cells, representing the most common ocular malignancy of childhood (prevalence approximately 1/20,000). **Bilateral** cases typically have a strong family history, whereas unilateral cases are most often sporadic. Retinoblastoma affects males and females equally.

Further reading

Chapter 3: Genetics. In: Forrester JV, Dick AD, McMenamin PG, Roberts F, Pearlman E. *The Eye: Basic Sciences in Practice* (5th Edition). Elsevier (2021).

67. D.

During meiosis, the **shorter** the distance between the two genes, the **higher the likelihood** that they will be transmitted together.

Further reading

Chapter 3: Genetics. In: Forrester JV, Dick AD, McMenamin PG, Roberts F, Pearlman E. *The Eye: Basic Sciences in Practice* (5th Edition). Elsevier (2021).

68. C.

On a pedigree chart, square boxes indicate male sex and circles indicate female sex. Solid shapes indicate affected individuals, half-shaded shapes indicate heterozygosity for recessive allele (i.e. carriers), and empty shapes indicate unaffected individuals. Fig. 4.1 displays pedigree charts for autosomal dominant and autosomal recessive inheritance. Fig. 4.2 is a key to explain common symbols used in pedigree charts.

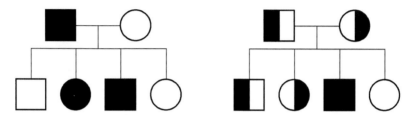

Figure 4.1 Pedigree charts for autosomal dominant (left) and autosomal recessive (right) inheritance.

Figure courtesy of Mr Umar Ahmed, Medical Student, Imperial College London.

	Male	Female	Sex unknown
Individual	□	○	◇
Affected individual	■	●	◆
Deceased	(slashed square)	(slashed circle)	(slashed diamond)
Pregnancy	P	P	P
Person providing pedigree information	□	○	◇

Figure 4.2 Pedigree chart key.

Figure courtesy of Mr Umar Ahmed, Medical Student, Imperial College London.

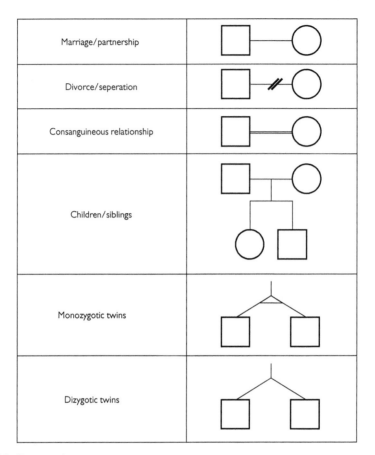

Marriage/partnership	
Divorce/seperation	
Consanguineous relationship	
Children/siblings	
Monozygotic twins	
Dizygotic twins	

Figure 4.2 Continued

Further reading

Chapter 3: Genetics. In: Forrester JV, Dick AD, McMenamin PG, Roberts F, Pearlman E. *The Eye: Basic Sciences in Practice* (5th Edition). Elsevier (2021).

Investigations 4

69. C.

This is a computed tomography angiogram demonstrating normal orbital anatomy, annotated in Fig. 4.3, which displays coronal and axial planes.

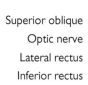
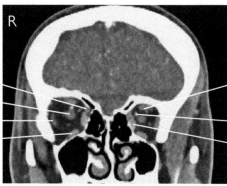

Superior oblique

Optic nerve

Lateral rectus

Inferior rectus

Superior rectus
& levator palpebrae
superioris

Ophthalmic artery

Medial rectus

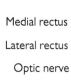
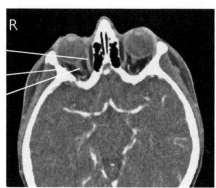

Medial rectus

Lateral rectus

Optic nerve

Figure 4.3 Basic orbital anatomy on a computed tomography angiogram, coronal plane (top) and axial plane (bottom). R = right side.

Figure courtesy of Mr Aswin Chari, Clinical Research Fellow in Neurosurgery, Great Ormond Street Hospital for Children, London.

Further reading

Mollan SP, Calcagni A, Keane PA. Chapter 2: Investigations and their interpretation. In: Denniston AKO, Murray PI. *Oxford Handbook of Ophthalmology*. Oxford University Press (2018).

70. D.

According to Traquair's analogy, the visual field is 'an island of vision surrounded by a sea of darkness'. Following this analogy, the fovea represents the peak of the 'hill'. At 'ground level', the visual field extends 50° superiorly, 60° nasally, 70° inferiorly, and 90° temporally.

Further reading

Mollan SP, Calcagni A, Keane PA. Chapter 2: Investigations and their interpretation. In: Denniston AKO, Murray PI. *Oxford Handbook of Ophthalmology*. Oxford University Press (2018).

71. D.

Pattern standard deviation (PSD) is a measure of variability or focal loss within the visual field. PSD takes into account any generalised depression. Therefore, a high PSD is more indicative of glaucomatous field loss than mean deviation, which is simply a measure of overall field loss.

Further reading

Mollan SP, Calcagni A, Keane PA. Chapter 2: Investigations and their interpretation. In: Denniston AKO, Murray PI. *Oxford Handbook of Ophthalmology*. Oxford University Press (2018).

72. B.

Colour fundus photography can be used in the diagnosis, screening, and monitoring of posterior segment disease. The optical field of view is typically 30° or 35°. Thus, they are not designed to image the peripheral retina. This renders colour fundus photography less useful in the early diagnosis of peripheral retinal tears or other conditions affecting the peripheral retina.

Further reading

Mollan SP, Calcagni A, Keane PA. Chapter 2: Investigations and their interpretation. In: Denniston AKO, Murray PI. *Oxford Handbook of Ophthalmology*. Oxford University Press (2018).

73. C.

In fundus fluorescein angiography, a window defect is most likely to be caused by a defect in the retinal pigment epithelium (RPE), e.g. macular hole or RPE atrophy.

Further reading

Mollan SP, Calcagni A, Keane PA. Chapter 2: Investigations and their interpretation. In: Denniston AKO, Murray PI. *Oxford Handbook of Ophthalmology*. Oxford University Press (2018).

74. C.

In false-colour display of OCT imaging, hyporeflective tissue is blue-black while hyperreflective tissue is reddish white. In greyscale display, hyporeflective tissue is dark grey while hyperreflective tissue is light grey. The ganglion cell layer and inner and outer nuclear layers are typically hyporeflective, while the nerve fibre layer and inner and outer plexiform layers are typically hyperreflective.

Further reading

Mollan SP, Calcagni A, Keane PA. Chapter 2: Investigations and their interpretation. In: Denniston AKO, Murray PI. *Oxford Handbook of Ophthalmology*. Oxford University Press (2018).

75. B.

Cystoid macular oedema (CMO) is characterised by intraretinal cystoid spaces filled with clear fluid and is likely caused by disruption of the blood–retinal barrier. A macular hole is a small break/opening in the macula. Soft drusen are small yellow-white dome-shaped deposits under the retinal pigment epithelium (RPE), associated with dry age-related macular degeneration (AMD). Geographic atrophy is an advanced form of dry AMD associated with atrophy of the outer retina, RPE, and choriocapillaris, leading to permanent loss in vision.

Further reading

Mollan SP, Calcagni A, Keane PA. Chapter 2: Investigations and their interpretation. In: Denniston AKO, Murray PI. *Oxford Handbook of Ophthalmology*. Oxford University Press (2018).

76. C.

In ocular ultrasonography, the gain control can adjust the **amplification of the reflected signal**. It does not change the amount of ultrasonic energy emitted from the probe.

Further reading

Mollan SP, Calcagni A, Keane PA. Chapter 2: Investigations and their interpretation. In: Denniston AKO, Murray PI. *Oxford Handbook of Ophthalmology*. Oxford University Press (2018).

77. D.

On A-scan, choroidal melanomas typically show medium to low internal reflectivity. On B-scan, choroidal melanomas most commonly appear dome-shaped; other characteristics include an acoustically hollow zone within the melanoma, subretinal fluid, and choroidal excavation. Optic disc drusen can be diagnosed on B-scan due to their high reflectivity; calcified drusen maintain high signal intensity even when the gain is reduced. The B-scan features of posterior scleritis include well-defined, thickened sclera and fluid in Tenon's space. Intraocular foreign bodies may also be detected on B-scan.

Further reading

Mollan SP, Calcagni A, Keane PA. Chapter 2: Investigations and their interpretation. In: Denniston AKO, Murray PI. *Oxford Handbook of Ophthalmology.* Oxford University Press (2018).

78. D.

The rod-response ERG obtained after dark adaptation (20 minutes in the dark) is achieved using a dim white flash below cone sensitivity—this comprises a b-wave only. The maximal ERG obtained from dark-adapted eyes using a bright white flash is a mixed rod and cone response.

Further reading

e-Learning for Healthcare. Eye-Site 12—neurophysiology. Available via: https://www.e-lfh.org.uk/pro grammes/ophthalmology/ Accessed November 2021.

McCulloch DL, Marmor MF, Brigell MG, et al. ISCEV Standard for full-field clinical electroretinography (2015 update). *Documenta Ophthalmologica. Advances in Ophthalmology.* 2015 Feb;*130*(1):1–12.

79. B.

The following conditions can reduce a- and b-waves: **R**od-cone dystrophies (including retinitis pigmentosa), **O**phthalmic artery occlusion, **D**rug toxicity (e.g. phenothiazines), **C**ancer-associated retinopathy, total **R**etinal detachment, **A**utoimmune retinopathy, **M**etallosis. These can be remembered using the acronym, '**ROD CRAM**'. X-linked retinoschisis can cause a normal a-wave and reduced scotopic b-wave, also termed an 'electronegative' response.

Further reading

Mollan SP, Calcagni A, Keane PA. Chapter 2: Investigations and their interpretation. In: Denniston AKO, Murray PI. *Oxford Handbook of Ophthalmology.* Oxford University Press (2018).

Miscellaneous 4

80. B.

Absolute risk reduction (ARR) describes the difference between the probability of an event occurring in two groups. This can be calculated as control event rate minus experimental event rate. The number needed to treat (NNT) is the number of people that must be treated for one beneficial event to occur. The number needed to harm (NNH) is the number of people that must be treated in order for one harmful event to occur. Both NNT and NNH are the reciprocal of ARR, i.e. NNT = 1/ARR.

Further reading

Denniston AKO, Moseley M, Murray PI. Chapter 26: Evidence-based ophthalmology. In: Denniston AKO, Murray PI. *Oxford Handbook of Ophthalmology.* Oxford University Press (2018).

81. C.

A Forest plot (or 'blobbogram') is used to display estimated results from several studies plus the overall meta-analysed measure of effect, which is represented by the dashed vertical line. The overall meta-analysed effect can also be plotted as a diamond whose lateral points indicate the confidence intervals. The solid vertical line represents the line of no effect. The size of the boxes indicates the individual study power (and therefore sample size) while the horizontal 'whiskers' indicate the confidence intervals per individual study.

Further reading

Denniston AKO, Moseley M, Murray PI. Chapter 26: Evidence-based ophthalmology. In: Denniston AKO, Murray PI. *Oxford Handbook of Ophthalmology*. Oxford University Press (2018).

82. B.

Fig. 4.4 summarizes the data points displayed on a box and whisker plot. Please note that box and whisker plots can be orientated horizontally or vertically.

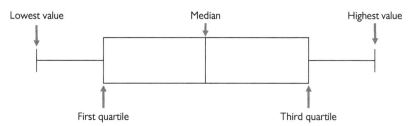

Figure 4.4 The box and whisker plot.

© Sohaib R. Rufai 2021.

Further reading

Bunce C, Young-Zvandasara T. Simplified Ophthalmic Statistics (SOS). Part 2: How to summarise your data and why it's a good idea to do so. *Eye News*. 2018;25(2):34–35. Available at: https://www.eyenews.uk.com/education/trainees/post/sos-simplified-ophthalmic-statistics-part-2-how-to-summarise-your-data-and-why-it-s-a-good-idea-to-do-so Accessed October 2021.

83. C.

The World Health Organization recommends the ICD-11 definitions for distance and near visual impairment.

Distance visual impairment:

- Mild: visual acuity worse than 6/12 to 6/18.
- Moderate: visual acuity worse than 6/18 to 6/60.
- Severe: visual acuity worse than 6/60 to 3/60.
- Blindness: visual acuity worse than 3/60.

Near visual impairment:

- Near visual acuity worse than N6 or M.08 at 40 cm.

Further reading

World Health Organization. Blindness and vision impairment. 14 October 2021. Available at: https://www.who.int/news-room/fact-sheets/detail/blindness-and-visual-impairment Accessed October 2021.

84. D.

According to the World Health Organization, at least 2.2 billion people worldwide have a near or distance visual impairment. In at least 1 billion, visual impairment either could have been prevented or is yet to be addressed. The leading causes of visual impairment globally are uncorrected refractive errors, cataract, age-related macular degeneration, glaucoma, diabetic retinopathy, corneal opacity, and trachoma.

Further reading

World Health Organization. Blindness and vision impairment. 14 October 2021. Available at: https://www.who.int/news-room/fact-sheets/detail/blindness-and-visual-impairment Accessed October 2021.

85. A.

Fig. 1.10 (see p. xxx) is a flowchart displaying common statistical tests and rules.

Further reading

Bunce C, Young-Zvandasara T. Simplified Ophthalmic Statistics (SOS). Part 3: Which statistical test should I use (if any)? *Eye News.* 2019;25(4):34–36. Available at: https://www.eyenews.uk.com/education/trainees/post/sos-simplified-ophthalmic-statistics-part-3-which-statistical-test-should-i-use-if-any Accessed November 2021.

86. A.

Fig. 1.10 (see p. xxx) is a flowchart displaying common statistical tests and rules.

Further reading

Bunce C, Young-Zvandasara T. Simplified Ophthalmic Statistics (SOS). Part 3: Which statistical test should I use (if any)? *Eye News.* 2019;25(4):34–36. Available at: https://www.eyenews.uk.com/education/trainees/post/sos-simplified-ophthalmic-statistics-part-3-which-statistical-test-should-i-use-if-any Accessed November 2021.

87. A.

Attrition bias can result due to unequal loss of participants from different arms of a trial. Selection bias can be caused by failure to achieve proper randomisation during participant selection. Confirmation bias can be caused by the tendency to search for or favour information that confirms prior beliefs. Recall bias can be caused by differences in the accuracy or completeness of recollections by participants regarding past events.

Further reading

Denniston AKO, Moseley M, Murray PI. Chapter 26: Evidence-based ophthalmology. In: Denniston AKO, Murray PI. *Oxford Handbook of Ophthalmology.* Oxford University Press (2018).

88.

   I. C.
   II. A.
   III. B.

Equations for diagnostic accuracy testing:

$$Sensitivity = \frac{TP}{TP + FN}$$

$$Specificity = \frac{TN}{TN + FP}$$

$$PPV = \frac{TP}{TP + FP}$$

$$NPV = \frac{TN}{TN + FN}$$

$$Positive\ likelihood\ ratio = \frac{sensitivity}{1 - specificity}$$

$$Negative\ likelihood\ ratio = \frac{1 - sensitivity}{specificity}$$

$$Accuracy = \frac{TP + TN}{TP + TN + FP + FN}$$

Further reading

Denniston AKO, Moseley M, Murray PI. Chapter 26: Evidence-based ophthalmology. In: Denniston AKO, Murray PI. *Oxford Handbook of Ophthalmology*. Oxford University Press (2018).

Optics 5

1. **A visual acuity of 0.3 logMAR is equivalent to which of the following on the Snellen chart?**
   A. 6/9
   B. 6/12
   C. 6/18
   D. 6/24

2. **Which of the following clinical tests of stereoacuity require red–green spectacles?**
   A. Lang
   B. Frisby
   C. TNO
   D. Titmus

3. **Regarding the refractive index, which statement is LEAST likely to be correct?**
   A. Absolute refractive index = velocity of light in vacuum/velocity of light in medium.
   B. The refractive index of air is 1.
   C. A refractometer can determine the absolute refractive index of a material.
   D. Light is deviated away from the normal on entering an optically dense medium from a less dense medium.

4. **Which of the following does NOT determine the angle of deviation for a prism in air:**
   A. The refractive index of the material of which the prism is composed
   B. The angle of incidence of the ray considered
   C. The circle of least confusion
   D. The refracting angle of the prism

MCQs for FRCOphth Part 1. Sohaib R. Rufai, Oxford University Press. © Oxford University Press 2023.
DOI: 10.1093/oso/9780192843715.003.0005

5. **Regarding vergence, which statement is LEAST likely to be correct?**
    A. Lenses of longer focal length are less powerful than lenses of shorter focal length.
    B. The unit of lens power is the dioptre.
    C. Diverging lenses can be used to correct myopia.
    D. Vergence power is based on the reciprocal of the first focal length.

6. **Which of the following best defines the Jackson cross cylinder?**
    A. A sphero-cylindrical lens wherein the power of the cylinder is half the power of the sphere and of the same sign
    B. A sphero-cylindrical lens wherein the power of the cylinder is half the power of the sphere and of the opposite sign
    C. A sphero-cylindrical lens wherein the power of the cylinder is twice the power of the sphere and of the same sign
    D. A sphero-cylindrical lens wherein the power of the cylinder is twice the power of the sphere and of the opposite sign

7. **Regarding reducing ocular spherical aberration, which of the following statements is LEAST likely to be correct?**
    A. The cornea and lens form an aplanatic surface.
    B. The iris acts as a stop to reduce spherical aberration.
    C. The lens cortex has a higher refractive index than the lens nucleus.
    D. Cone photoreceptors are more sensitive to light entering the eye paraxially as opposed to light entering obliquely through peripheral cornea.

8. **Which of the Purkinje–Sanson images is a real, inverted image?**
    A. I
    B. II
    C. III
    D. IV

9. **Regarding myopia, which statement is LEAST likely to be correct?**
    A. In the myopic eye, the second principal focus lies in front of the retina.
    B. In axial myopia, the eye is abnormally long.
    C. Axial and refractive myopia can occur in keratoconus.
    D. In nuclear sclerosis, the refractive power of the lens decreases as the nucleus becomes more dense.

10. **Regarding the effective power of lenses, which statement is MOST likely to be true?**
    A. If the correcting lens is moved towards a hypermetropic eye, the effectivity of the lens is increased.
    B. In uncorrected myopia, the image falls behind the retina.
    C. If the correcting lens is moved away from a myopic eye, then a stronger concave lens is required to throw the image onto the retina.
    D. Back vertex distance is the distance between the pupil and the back of the correcting lens.

11. **In presbyopia, how much of the available accommodation must be kept in reserve to permit comfortable near vision?**
    A. 1/5
    B. 1/4
    C. 1/3
    D. 1/2

12. **Regarding optical problems associated with contact lens wear, which statement is LEAST likely to be correct?**
    A. Contact lenses may move excessively on blinking if the posterior contact lens surface is too flat.
    B. Corneal warpage is more pronounced with rigid contact lenses as opposed to soft contact lenses.
    C. Corneal warpage describes the change in corneal curvature that is not associated with corneal oedema.
    D. Contact lenses increase the aniseikonia associated with anisometropia.

13. **What are the characteristics of the image produced by indirect ophthalmoscopy, as studied by the observer?**
    A. Virtual, horizontally inverted
    B. Virtual, horizontally and vertically inverted
    C. Real, horizontally inverted
    D. Real, horizontally and vertically inverted

14. **Regarding Placido's disc, which statement is MOST likely to be true?**
    A. A concave lens is mounted in the central aperture.
    B. Best results are achieved by placing a bright light source in front of the patient's eye.
    C. In an astigmatic patient, the rings appear closer in the steeper meridian.
    D. The shorter the radius of curvature of the anterior corneal surface, the wider apart the rings of the Placido disc.

15. **Regarding the slit lamp, which statement is MOST likely to be true?**
    A. It comprises two relatively high-powered compound microscopes.
    B. The compound microscopes and lighting system possess a common focal plane.
    C. The microscope has relatively short working distances.
    D. Diffuse illumination involves focusing a wide slit beam directly upon the part of the eye to be inspected.

16. **Regarding specular microscopy, which statement is LEAST likely to be true?**
    A. Specular microscopy is used to assess the suitability of donor corneas.
    B. Reflection from the corneal surface is reduced by direct contact of the instrument to the cornea.
    C. Specular reflections arise from light reflected by structures of similar refractive indices.
    D. Specular microscopy can be used to assess hexagonal cell ratio.

Anatomy 5

17. Regarding the superior orbital fissure, which statement is MOST likely to be true?

A. The superior orbital fissure lies between the roof and medial walls of the orbit.

B. Its widest part is at its lateral end.

C. From lateral to medial, the trochlear nerve, frontal nerve, and lacrimal nerve pass through the superior orbital fissure outside the annulus of Zinn.

D. There exists a small, sharp spine for the lateral rectus muscle approximately halfway on the lower edge of the superior orbital fissure.

18. What is the correct order of eyelid constituents, from superficial to deep?

A. Skin, subcutaneous tissue, orbital septum and tarsal plates, striated muscle fibres of orbicularis oculi, smooth muscle, conjunctiva

B. Skin, subcutaneous tissue, striated muscle fibres of orbicularis oculi, orbital septum and tarsal plates, smooth muscle, conjunctiva

C. Skin, subcutaneous tissue, striated muscle fibres of orbicularis oculi, conjunctiva, smooth muscle, orbital septum, and tarsal plates

D. Skin, subcutaneous tissue, smooth muscle, striated muscle fibres of orbicularis oculi, orbital septum and tarsal plates, conjunctiva

19. The visual axis forms a line connecting which two parts of the eye?

A. The fovea centralis and the nodal point

B. The optic nerve and the anterior pole

C. The posterior pole and the nodal point

D. The posterior pole and the anterior pole

20. What proportion of the eyeball is formed by the sclera?

A. 1/2

B. 3/4

C. 4/5

D. 5/6

21. Regarding the corneal epithelium, which statement is LEAST likely to be true?

A. The cells of the superficial layer are attached by desmosomes.

B. The cells of the middle zone are polyhedral in shape.

C. The basement membrane is weakly attached to Bowman's layer.

D. The basement membrane stains positive with periodic acid–Schiff.

22. **Which of the following structures is NOT found within the lateral wall of the cavernous sinus?**
   A. Trochlear nerve
   B. Maxillary division of trigeminal nerve
   C. Oculomotor nerve
   D. Abducens nerve

23. **Regarding the iris, which statement is LEAST likely to be true?**
   A. Its central pupillary zone and peripheral ciliary zone is separated by the collarette.
   B. Its stroma is derived from neuroectoderm.
   C. It is approximately 12 mm in diameter.
   D. Its anterior surface is devoid of epithelium.

24. **Regarding the retinal pigment epithelium (RPE), which statement is MOST likely to be true?**
   A. The RPE cells are tall and narrow near the ora serrata.
   B. The RPE cell nuclei are situated in the apical cytoplasm.
   C. The RPE cells are joined together by tight junctions.
   D. The RPE develops from the inner layer of the optic cup.

25. **What is the approximate volume of the anterior chamber of the eye, in millilitres (mL)?**
   A. 0.2 mL
   B. 0.4 mL
   C. 0.6 mL
   D. 0.8 mL

26. **Regarding the vitreous body, which statement is LEAST likely to be true?**
   A. Its centre is denser than its cortex.
   B. It consists of 98% water.
   C. The hyaloid canal is approximately 1–2 mm wide.
   D. The hyaloid artery disappears 6 weeks before birth.

27. **Which of the following muscle actions result in levoversion?**
   A. Contraction of both superior recti
   B. Contraction of both inferior recti
   C. Contraction of right lateral rectus and left medial rectus
   D. Contraction of right medial rectus and left lateral rectus

28. **Regarding the abducens nerve, which statement is MOST likely to be true?**

    A. It has the shortest intracranial course of all the cranial nerves.

    B. Its nucleus is situated in the mid-pons, beneath the floor of the upper part of the fourth ventricle.

    C. It emerges from the posterior surface of the brainstem.

    D. It passes through the superior orbital fissure outside the common tendinous ring.

29. **What are the approximate dimensions of the optic chiasm?**

    A. 8 mm wide and 4 mm long

    B. 10 mm wide and 6 mm long

    C. 12 mm wide and 8 mm long

    D. 14 mm wide and 10 mm long

30. **Which of the following ocular structures is NOT derived from surface ectoderm?**

    A. Corneal epithelium

    B. Sclera

    C. Lens

    D. Lacrimal gland

Physiology 5

Physiology of the eye and vision

31. **Regarding aqueous humour, which statement is MOST likely to be true?**

    A. In healthy eyes, an average intraocular pressure of approximately 10 mmHg is generated by the flow of aqueous humour against resistance.

    B. The refractive index of aqueous humour is 1.38.

    C. The concentration of ascorbate in aqueous humour is 20 times less than that in plasma.

    D. The concentration of protein in aqueous humour is 200 times less than that in plasma.

32. **Regarding protection of the human lens against oxidative damage, which statement is LEAST likely to be true?**

    A. Glutathione and glycine protect the lens against oxidative damage.

    B. Reduced glutathione is regenerated from oxidised glutathione reductase and reduced nicotinamide adenine dinucleotide phosphate (NADPH).

    C. The hexose monophosphate shunt is responsible for much of the NADPH production in the lens.

    D. Increased glutathione levels in lens epithelial cells cause cataract formation.

33. **At the end of which week of embryological development does the secondary vitreous appear?**
   A. Fourth
   B. Sixth
   C. Eighth
   D. Tenth

34. **Regarding transport across the retinal pigment epithelium (RPE), which statement is LEAST likely to be true?**
   A. Docosahexaenoic is synthesised by the photoreceptors.
   B. Glucose transporters GLUT1 and GLUT3 are abundant in the apical and basolateral membrane.
   C. Water and lactic acid are removed from the subretinal space via active transcellular transport by the RPE.
   D. Tight junctions of the RPE cells form the outer blood–retinal barrier.

35. **Regarding the accommodative mechanism, which statement is MOST likely to be true?**
   A. When the ciliary muscle relaxes, the lens capsule moulds the young lens into a more spherical form.
   B. The increase in curvature of the lens' posterior surface increases the optical power of the lens.
   C. During accommodation, the thickness of the lens nucleus does not change.
   D. The Helmholtz accommodative mechanism did not describe anterior movement of the anterior lens surface.

36. **Which wavelength are short-wavelength-sensitive (S) cone photopigments most sensitive to, in nanometres (nm)?**
   A. 560 nm
   B. 530 nm
   C. 415 nm
   D. 380 nm

General physiology

37. **Regarding skeletal muscle, which statement is LEAST likely to be true?**
   A. The surface layer of the sarcolemma fuses with a tendon fibre at each end of the muscle fibre.
   B. Titin filamentous molecules form a framework, holding the myosin and actin filaments in place.
   C. Each myofibril is composed of approximately 1500 myosin filaments and 3000 actin filaments.
   D. Sarcoplasm contains large quantities of potassium and small quantities of magnesium and phosphate.

38. **Regarding synaptic transmission at the neuromuscular junction, which statement is MOST likely to be true?**

    A. When an action potential reaches the neuromuscular junction, voltage-gated sodium channels are activated.
    B. Calcium/calmodulin-dependent protein kinase phosphorylates synapsin proteins that anchor acetylcholine vesicles to the presynaptic terminal.
    C. Acetylcholine vesicles fuse with the neural membrane and release acetylcholine into the synaptic cleft via endocytosis.
    D. Neostigmine stimulates the neuromuscular junction by activating acetylcholinesterase.

39. **Regarding the pancreas, which statement is LEAST likely to be true?**

    A. The pancreas contains 4–6 million islets of Langerhans.
    B. The acini secrete digestive juices directly into the ileum.
    C. The delta cells secrete amylin.
    D. The alpha cells comprise 25% of the islets of Langerhans.

40. **Regarding vitamin deficiencies, which statement is LEAST likely to be correct?**

    A. Vitamin A deficiency causes night blindness.
    B. Vitamin B_1 deficiency causes gastrointestinal tract disturbances.
    C. Vitamin B_{12} deficiency causes cardiac failure.
    D. Vitamin C deficiency causes scurvy.

Biochemistry

41. **Regarding mitochondria, which statement is MOST likely to be true?**

    A. They are approximately 8 micrometres long.
    B. They comprise a three-membrane system of compartments.
    C. The mitochondrion outer membrane organising system is located at the cristae junction with the outer boundary membrane.
    D. Proteins in the inner boundary membrane assist in protein movement.

42. **Regarding matrix factors affecting corneal transparency, which statement is MOST likely to be true?**

    A. The stroma accounts for approximately 55% of total corneal thickness.
    B. Type I collagen accounts for approximately 90% of stromal collagen.
    C. Stromal type I collagen is arranged in parallel.
    D. Types I, III, and V collagen are fibrillary collagens.

43. Regarding the biochemical changes observed in cataract formation, which statement is LEAST likely to be true?

A. The ordered packing of lens crystallins is disturbed by increased water accumulation in the lens.

B. Ultraviolet B (UV-B) light exposure is associated with an increase in nuclear cataract formation.

C. Water clefts in the lens are suggestive of reduced function of aquaporin-0 (AQP0) and fluid transport.

D. In nuclear cataract formation, there is significant oxidation of cystine and methionine residues on lens proteins.

Pathology 5

General and ocular pathology

44. Regarding cell death, which statement is LEAST likely to be true?

A. Necrosis is always pathological.

B. Necrosis is typically associated with an inflammatory reaction.

C. Apoptosis usually affects single cells within a population of healthy cells.

D. Apoptosis is a passive process involving cleavage of proteins by caspase enzymes.

45. Regarding neoplasia, which statement is MOST likely to be correct?

A. The growth of a neoplasm halts after the initiating stimulus has been withdrawn.

B. Malignant neoplasms are often slow growing.

C. Benign neoplasms typically have ill-defined boundaries.

D. Benign neoplasms may undergo malignant transformation.

46. Which of the following pathological processes does NOT occur in age-related macular degeneration?

A. Reduced production of extracellular matrix.

B. Accumulation of lipofuscin in the retinal pigment epithelium.

C. Sub-retinal pigment epithelium deposit formation with associated photoreceptor cell death.

D. Metabolic and phagocytic insufficiency of retinal pigment epithelium.

47. Which human leukocyte antigen (HLA) is most likely to be associated with Behçet's retinal vasculitis?

A. HLA-B51

B. HLA-DR4

C. HLA-B27

D. HLA-A29

48. Regarding secondary glaucoma, which statement is MOST likely to be true?

A. Posterior synechiae are adhesions that form between the peripheral iris and trabecular meshwork.

B. In neovascular glaucoma, adhesions are formed between the iris and trabecular meshwork due to rubeotic fibrovascular proliferation.

C. Pseudoexfoliation syndrome is the most common form of secondary closed-angle glaucoma.

D. Secondary open-angle glaucoma is caused by the mechanical closure of the iridocorneal angle due to anterior displacement of the lens.

49. Regarding lattice corneal dystrophy, which statement is MOST likely to be true?

A. It is inherited in an autosomal recessive manner.

B. Clinically, it is characterised by fine lines criss-crossing the stroma.

C. Microscopy reveals lipofuscin deposits.

D. It rarely recurs in corneal grafts.

50. Regarding optic pathway gliomas, which statement is LEAST likely to be true?

A. Adult forms carry a good prognosis.

B. Gliomas involving the orbital portion of the optic nerve can be associated with proptosis, papilloedema, and loss of vision.

C. Excised gliomas demonstrate a fusiform swelling of the nerve.

D. The prevalence of optic pathway gliomas in patients with neurofibromatosis type 1 is approximately 15–25%.

51. Regarding eyelid cysts, which statement is MOST likely to be true?

A. Dermoid cysts originate from the glands of Moll.

B. Sudoriferous cysts can occur due to epithelial inclusion following trauma.

C. Epidermoid cysts contain pilosebaceous follicles and hair.

D. Hidrocystomas are lined by a double layer of epithelium.

52. Regarding lacrimal gland tumours, which statement is LEAST likely to be true?

A. Pleomorphic adenoma represents the most common epithelial tumour of the lacrimal gland.

B. Histologically, adenoid cystic carcinomas most commonly assume a cribriform or 'Swiss-cheese' pattern.

C. Mucoepidermoid carcinoma may arise in the lacrimal gland.

D. Lacrimal sac tumours do not tend to invade surrounding structures.

Microbiology

53. Which of the following organisms is LEAST likely to represent normal ocular flora?

A. *Staphylococcus epidermis*

B. *Staphylococcus aureus*

C. *Cutibacterium acnes* (formerly *Propionibacterium acnes*)

D. *Bacillus cereus*

54. Regarding ocular fungal pathogens, which statement is LEAST likely to be true?

A. *Aspergillus* spp. and *Candida* spp. can directly invade the cornea and anterior segment.

B. Mucormycosis commonly occurs in immunocompetent individuals.

C. *Mucor* spp. can parasitise the ophthalmic artery and its branches.

D. Histoplasmosis is more prevalent in the United States as compared to the United Kingdom.

Immunology

55. Which of the following characteristics is NOT inherent to the acquired immune response?

A. Memory

B. Diversity

C. Ability to downregulate

D. Rapid mobilisation

56. Regarding cytokines, which statement is MOST likely to be true?

A. They demonstrate pleiotropism.

B. They are short-lived and long-range molecules.

C. They are only effective in high concentrations.

D. They cannot alter the effects of other cytokines.

Pharmacology and genetics 5

Pharmacology

57. Which of the following drugs does NOT act as a microsomal enzyme inducer?

A. Phenytoin

B. Warfarin

C. Rifampicin

D. Nicotine

58. **To which class of intraocular pressure-lowering drugs does pilocarpine belong?**

    A. α_2-adrenostimulants
    B. Parasympathomimetics
    C. Carbonic anhydrase inhibitors
    D. Prostaglandin analogues

59. **Which of the following is LEAST likely to represent an ocular side effect of topical steroids?**

    A. Reactivation of viral keratitis
    B. Cataract formation
    C. Increased incidence of bacterial infection
    D. Acute angle-closure glaucoma

60. **Which of the following is MOST likely to represent a side effect of azathioprine?**

    A. Bone marrow suppression
    B. Nephrotoxicity
    C. Osteoporosis
    D. Hypertension

61. **Which of the following is MOST likely to be associated with Horner's syndrome?**

    A. Increased sweating to affected side of face
    B. Loss of sympathetic tone to iris
    C. Complete ptosis
    D. Inferior pulmonary sulcus tumour

62. **Regarding pharmacological diagnosis of Horner's syndrome, which of the following drops prevents the reuptake of noradrenaline?**

    A. Apraclonidine
    B. Phenylephrine
    C. Hydroxyamphetamine
    D. Cocaine

Genetics

63. **Which of the following nucleotide bases is NOT present in messenger RNA (mRNA)?**

    A. Guanine
    B. Thymine
    C. Adenine
    D. Cytosine

64. **Regarding translation, which statement is LEAST likely to be true?**
    A. The stop codon on the messenger RNA causes binding of release factor to the peptidyl-tRNA-binding site (P site).
    B. Aminoacyl-tRNA synthetases couple amino acids to the appropriate transfer RNA molecule.
    C. Peptidyl transferase is present on the ribosome.
    D. The polypeptide chain is produced from the N-terminal end to the C-terminal end.

65. **Which of the following is NOT characteristic of autosomal dominant inheritance?**
    A. Vertical transmission
    B. Constant expressivity
    C. Homozygotes most severely affected
    D. 50% of offspring affected

66. **Regarding epigenetics, which statement is LEAST likely to be true?**
    A. Genetic imprinting is different from both father and mother.
    B. Cancer may be caused by alteration in DNA methylation patterns.
    C. Genetic imprinting results from heritable patterns.
    D. An epigenetic trait results from changes in a chromosome, thus altering the DNA sequence.

67. **Which of the following gene mutations is NOT associated with Stargardt disease?**
    A. *ABCA4*
    B. *COL2A1*
    C. *ELOVL4*
    D. *RDS*

68. **Regarding twin studies, which statement is MOST likely to be true?**
    A. Continuous traits either demonstrate severe disease expression or no expression.
    B. Multifactorial discontinuous traits demonstrate increased incidence in the general population compared to affected families.
    C. In multifactorial inheritance, the incidence of the trait in dizygotic twins is lower than that in monozygotic twins.
    D. Discontinuous multifactorial traits demonstrate equal sex distribution.

Investigations 5

69. **In Humphrey perimetry, which of the following is MOST likely to lead to a high false-positive rate?**
    A. The patient moves during testing
    B. The patient becomes tired during testing
    C. The patient presses the response button too often
    D. The light stimulus stops working mid-way through testing

70. **Regarding Goldmann perimetry interpretation, what do the Roman numerals represent?**
    A. Intensity of light in apostilbs
    B. Size of the target in mm^2
    C. Additional minor light filters
    D. Visual field quadrants

71. **Regarding fundus fluorescein angiography, which statement is MOST likely to be true?**
    A. Sodium fluorescein is insoluble in water.
    B. Fluorescein is stimulated by 530 nm light and emits 490 nm light.
    C. Fluorescein is metabolised by the liver and excreted by the kidneys.
    D. Sodium fluorescein is 30% bound to plasma albumin.

72. **In fundus fluorescein angiography (FFA), which of the following conditions is LEAST likely to cause leakage of dye?**
    A. Cystoid macular oedema
    B. Papilloedema
    C. Choroidal neovascularisation
    D. Retinal pigment epithelium atrophy

73. **What axial resolution can be achieved in spectral domain optical coherence tomography (OCT)?**
    A. 3–8 micrometres
    B. 9–12 micrometres
    C. 13–16 micrometres
    D. 17–20 micrometres

74. Regarding the optical coherence tomography (OCT) image of the optic nerve head displayed below, what is the MOST likely diagnosis?

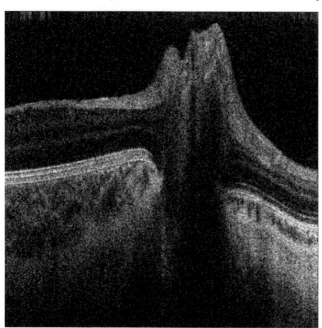

Adapted from: Rufai SR, et al. Feasibility and Repeatability of Handheld Optical Coherence Tomography in Children with Craniosynostosis. *Transl Vis Sci Technol.* 2021 Jul 1;10(8):24.

A. Optic atrophy
B. Papilloedema
C. Primary open-angle glaucoma
D. Tilted disc syndrome

75. Regarding scanning laser ophthalmoscopy (SLO), which statement is LEAST likely to be correct?

A. SLO generates higher-contrast images than standard fundus photography.
B. Light scatter is reduced in SLO because only a small area of the fundus is illuminated at any given time.
C. SLO devices use a confocal aperture.
D. SLO devices deliver higher spatial resolution than standard fundus cameras.

76. Which substance appears brighter on T2-weighted magnetic resonance imaging (MRI) as compared to T1-weighted MRI?

A. Air
B. Dense bone
C. Fat
D. Cerebrospinal fluid

77. **Regarding the full-field electroretinogram (ERG), the a-wave arises primarily from which of the following structures?**
    A. Amacrine cells
    B. Photoreceptors
    C. Müller cells
    D. Bipolar cells

78. **Regarding the electro-oculogram (EOG), what is the normal light peak:dark trough (LP:DT) ratio?**
    A. 0.7–3.3
    B. 1.7–4.3
    C. 2.7–5.3
    D. 3.7–6.3

79. **Regarding the pattern electroretinogram (PERG), which statement is MOST likely to be true?**
    A. It utilises a reversing chequerboard to evoke small potentials from the outer retina.
    B. A normal PERG features a prominent negative component at 50 milliseconds (P50).
    C. N95 originates from the macular ganglion cells.
    D. The N95/P50 ratio is typically greater than 2.

Miscellaneous 5

80. **According to the Scottish Intercollegiate Guidelines Network (SIGN) classification, which of the following represents the lowest level of evidence?**
    A. Case–control study
    B. Case series
    C. Cohort study
    D. Randomised controlled trial

81. **On a Forest plot, what do the horizontal whiskers represent?**
    A. Study power
    B. Overall meta-analysed measure of effect
    C. Line of no effect
    D. Confidence intervals

82. **What is the grey arrow on the following box and whisker plot MOST likely to represent?**

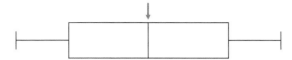

   A. Most commonly occurring data point
   B. Interquartile range
   C. Sum of all data points divided by two
   D. Middle point of a data set, when arranged in ascending order

83. **What is the definition of near visual impairment measured binocularly according to the International Classification of Diseases, 11th revision (ICD-11)?**
   A. Visual acuity worse than N6 at 40 cm
   B. Visual acuity worse than N5 at 40 cm
   C. Visual acuity worse than N6 at 30 cm
   D. Visual acuity worse than N5 at 30 cm

84. **In a study assessing whether adverse events are similar in one topical steroid medication compared to another, what is the MOST appropriate statistical test to use?**
   A. Fisher's exact test
   B. McNemar's test
   C. Kruskal–Wallis test
   D. Wilcoxon signed rank test

85. **What is the MOST appropriate statistical test to use for two groups where the outcome measure is continuous and the data are non-parametric and unpaired?**
   A. Chi-squared test
   B. Mann–Whitney U test
   C. Fisher's exact test
   D. Unpaired t-test

86. **Regarding the Kruskal–Wallis test, which statement is MOST likely to be correct?**
   A. It should be used where the outcome measure is categorical and the data are paired.
   B. It should be used where the outcome measure is categorical and the data are unpaired.
   C. It should be used where there are more than two groups and the data are parametric.
   D. It should be used where there are more than two groups and the data are non-parametric.

87. Which of the following options is MOST likely to lead to selection bias?

A. Differences in the accuracy or completeness of recollections by participants regarding past events.

B. The tendency to search for or favour information that confirms prior beliefs.

C. Failure to achieve proper randomisation during participant selection.

D. Unequal loss of participants from different arms of a trial.

88. Which of the following options correctly describes the main goal of a phase IV clinical trial?

A. Assessing pharmacokinetics

B. Assessing toxicity

C. Post-marketing surveillance in public

D. Dose-ranging for safety

89. Approximately how many human participants are recruited to a phase III clinical trial?

A. 10–20

B. 100–200

C. 300–3000

D. Over 3000

90. Regarding the preclinical phase of a clinical trial, which statement is LEAST likely to be correct?

A. Information on efficacy is gathered.

B. Information on toxicity is gathered.

C. The drug dose is not restricted.

D. Healthy human volunteers are tested.

Optics 5

1. B.

Table 5.1 shows conversions from logMAR visual acuities to Snellen equivalent.

Table 5.1 Conversions from logMAR visual acuities to Snellen equivalent

logMAR visual acuity	Snellen equivalent (metres)
1.00	6/60
0.90	6/48
0.80	6/38
0.70	6/30
0.60	6/24
0.50	6/19
0.40	6/15
0.30	6/12
0.20	6/9.5
0.10	6/7.5
0.00	6/6
−0.10	6/4.8
−0.20	6/3.8
−0.30	6/3

Further reading

Chapter 1: Clinical skills. In: Denniston AKO, Murray PI. *Oxford Handbook of Ophthalmology*. Oxford University Press (2018).

2. C.

The TNO test requires red-green spectacles. The Titmus test, which includes the Wirt fly test, requires polarising spectacles. The Lang and Frisby tests do not require any spectacles.

Further reading

Chapter 1: Properties of light and visual function. In: Elkington AR, Frank HJ, Greaney MJ. *Clinical Optics*. Blackwell Science (1999).

3. D.

Light is deviated **towards** from the normal on entering an optically dense medium from a less dense medium.

Further reading

Chapter 3: Refraction of light. In: Elkington AR, Frank HJ, Greaney MJ. *Clinical Optics*. Blackwell Science (1999).

4. C.

The circle of least confusion relates to toric lenses. Other options are true.

Further reading

Chapter 4: Prisms. In: Elkington AR, Frank HJ, Greaney MJ. *Clinical Optics*. Blackwell Science (1999).

5. D.

Vergence power is based on the reciprocal of the second focal length (f_2).

Further reading

Chapter 5: Spherical lenses. In: Elkington AR, Frank HJ, Greaney MJ. *Clinical Optics*. Blackwell Science (1999).

6. D.

The Jackson cross cylinder is a sphero-cylindrical lens wherein the power of the cylinder is twice the power of the sphere and of the same sign.

Further reading

Chapter 6: Astigmatic lenses. In: Elkington AR, Frank HJ, Greaney MJ. *Clinical Optics*. Blackwell Science (1999).

7. C.

The lens nucleus has a higher refractive index than the lens cortex, hence the axial zone of the lens possesses greater refractive power than the lens periphery. Other options are true. Option D is the Stiles–Crawford effect.

Further reading

Artal P, Tabernero J. The eye's aplanatic answer. *Nature Photonics*. 2008;2(10):586–589.

Chapter 8: Aberrations of optical systems including the eye. In: Elkington AR, Frank HJ, Greaney MJ. *Clinical Optics*. Blackwell Science (1999).

8. D.

Image IV is a real, inverted image as it is formed by the posterior lens surface, i.e. a concave reflecting surface. Images I–III are erect, virtual images as they are formed from the anterior corneal, posterior corneal, and anterior lens surfaces, respectively, i.e. convex reflective surfaces.

Further reading

Chapter 9: Refraction by the eye. In: Elkington AR, Frank HJ, Greaney MJ. *Clinical Optics*. Blackwell Science (1999).

9. D.

In nuclear sclerosis, the refractive power of the lens increases as the nucleus becomes more dense—this is an example of refractive or index myopia.

Further reading

Chapter 10: Optics of ametropia. In: Elkington AR, Frank HJ, Greaney MJ. *Clinical Optics*. Blackwell Science (1999).

10. C.

If the correcting lens is moved away from a hypermetropic eye, the effectivity of the lens is increased. In uncorrected myopia, the image falls in front of the retina. Back vertex distance is the distance between the cornea and the back of the correcting lens.

Further reading

Chapter 10: Optics of ametropia. In: Elkington AR, Frank HJ, Greaney MJ. *Clinical Optics*. Blackwell Science (1999).

11. C.

In presbyopia, one-third of the available accommodation must be kept in reserve to permit comfortable near vision. Convex lenses allow the presbyopic patient to achieve comfortable near vision.

Further reading

Chapter 11: Presbyopia. In: Elkington AR, Frank HJ, Greaney MJ. *Clinical Optics*. Blackwell Science (1999).

12. D.

Contact lenses reduce the aniseikonia associated with high degrees of astigmatism and anisometropia. Contact lenses can also eliminate or reduce the aberrations associated with spectacles for high refractive errors.

Further reading

Chapter 12: Contact lenses. In: Elkington AR, Frank HJ, Greaney MJ. *Clinical Optics*. Blackwell Science (1999).

13. D.

In indirect ophthalmoscopy, the image studied by the observer is real, and horizontally and vertically inverted.

Further reading

Chapter 14: Instruments. In: Elkington AR, Frank HJ, Greaney MJ. *Clinical Optics*. Blackwell Science (1999).

14. C.

A convex lens is mounted in the central aperture to magnify the image and avoid accommodation. Best results are actually achieved by placing a bright light source behind the patient's head, brightly illuminating the Placido disc and leaving the patient's eye in shadow. The shorter the radius of curvature of the anterior corneal surface, the closer together the rings of the Placido disc appear, because the reflected image is smaller.

Further reading

Chapter 14: Instruments. In: Elkington AR, Frank HJ, Greaney MJ. *Clinical Optics*. Blackwell Science (1999).

15. B.

The slit lamp consists of a relatively low-powered binocular microscope. The microscope has a relatively long working distance, which permits the use of optical devices such as condensing lenses and the removal of corneal foreign bodies. Diffuse illumination involves throwing the slit beam slightly out of focus across the structure to be inspected.

Further reading

Chapter 14: Instruments. In: Elkington AR, Frank HJ, Greaney MJ. *Clinical Optics*. Blackwell Science (1999).

16. C.

Specular reflections arise from light reflected by structures of different refractive indices; the greater the differences in refractive indices, the more pronounced the effect.

Further reading

Chapter 14: Instruments. In: Elkington AR, Frank HJ, Greaney MJ. *Clinical Optics*. Blackwell Science (1999).

Anatomy 5

17. D.

The superior orbital fissure lies between the lesser and greater wings of sphenoid. Its widest part is at its medial end. From lateral to medial, the **L**acrimal nerve, **F**rontal nerve and **T**rochlear nerve pass through the superior orbital fissure outside the annulus of Zinn, while those passing through the annulus of Zinn include the **S**uperior division of the oculomotor nerve, **A**bducens nerve, **N**asociliary branch of the ophthalmic nerve and **I**nferior Division of the oculomotor nerve—you can remember these using the mnemonic: '**L**ive **F**rankly **T**o **S**ee **A**bsolutely **N**o **I**nsult.'

Further reading

Chapter 1: Anatomy of the eye and orbit. In: Forrester JV, Dick AD, McMenamin PG, Roberts F, Pearlman E. *The Eye: Basic Sciences in Practice* (4th Edition). Elsevier (2016).

Chapter 3: The orbital cavity. In: Snell RS, Lemp MA. *Clinical Anatomy of the Eye* (2nd Edition). John Wiley and Sons (1998).

18. B.

In addition, the upper lid receives the insertion of levator palpebrae superioris.

Further reading

Chapter 5: The ocular appendages. In: Snell RS, Lemp MA. *Clinical Anatomy of the Eye* (2nd Edition). John Wiley and Sons (1998).

19. A.

The visual axis is a hypothetical line connecting the fovea centralis and the nodal point. The optical axis connects the posterior pole and anterior pole. The equator lies halfway between the two poles.

Further reading

Chapter 6: The eyeball. In: Snell RS, Lemp MA. *Clinical Anatomy of the Eye* (2nd Edition). John Wiley and Sons (1998).

20. **D.**

Five-sixths of the eyeball is formed by the opaque sclera, while one-sixth is formed by the transparent cornea.

Further reading

Chapter 6: The eyeball. In: Snell RS, Lemp MA. *Clinical Anatomy of the Eye* (2nd Edition). John Wiley and Sons (1998).

21. **C.**

The basement membrane is strongly attached to Bowman's layer. Other responses are true.

Further reading

Chapter 6: The eyeball. In: Snell RS, Lemp MA. *Clinical Anatomy of the Eye* (2nd Edition). John Wiley and Sons (1998).

22. **D.**

The following structures are found within the lateral wall of the cavernous sinus, from superior to inferior: oculomotor nerve, trochlear nerve, ophthalmic division of trigeminal nerve, and maxillary division of trigeminal nerve. The internal carotid artery and abducens nerve pass through the cavernous sinus.

Further reading

Chapter 1: An overview of the anatomy of the skull. In: Snell RS, Lemp MA. *Clinical Anatomy of the Eye* (2nd Edition). John Wiley and Sons (1998)

23. **B.**

The anteriorly situated stroma is derived from mesoderm while the two posteriorly situated epithelial layers are derived from neuroectoderm. Fig. 5.1 displays basic iris anatomy.

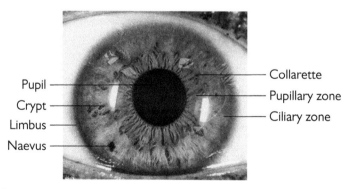

Figure 5.1 Basic iris anatomy.

Image courtesy of Mr Dermot F. Roche, Vision Scientist, Great Ormond Street Hospital for Children, London, with special thanks to Dr Tania Aslam Rufai, GP Registrar, Kent, UK.

Further reading

Chapter 6: The eyeball. In: Snell RS, Lemp MA. *Clinical Anatomy of the Eye* (2nd Edition). John Wiley and Sons (1998).

24. C.

The RPE cells are tall and narrow in the posterior pole and flattened near the ora serrata. The cell nuclei are situated in the basal cytoplasm. The RPE develops from the outer layer of the optic cup.

Further reading

Chapter 6: The eyeball. In: Snell RS, Lemp MA. *Clinical Anatomy of the Eye* (2nd Edition). John Wiley and Sons (1998).

25. A.

The volume of the anterior chamber of the eye is approximately 0.2 mL. Please note that this value differs slightly between sources.

Further reading

Chapter 6: The eyeball. In: Snell RS, Lemp MA. *Clinical Anatomy of the Eye* (2nd Edition). John Wiley and Sons (1998).

26. A.

The vitreous has a more liquid centre and denser base. From adolescence, the vitreous undergoes liquefaction starting in its centre and progressing further with age. This age-related change may predispose to vitreous detachment and/or retinal detachment.

Further reading

Chapter 6: The eyeball. In: Snell RS, Lemp MA. *Clinical Anatomy of the Eye* (2nd Edition). John Wiley and Sons (1998).

27. D.

'Dextroversion' describes both eyes turning to the right, while 'levoversion' describes both eyes turning to the left (from that person's perspective, as opposed to an onlooker's perspective). Similarly, 'supraversion' describes upward gaze, while 'infraversion' describes downward gaze. 'Dextrocycloversion' describes rightward rotation of the eyes, while 'levocycloversion' describes leftward rotation of the eyes.

Further reading

Chapter 8: Movements of the eyeball and the extraocular muscles. In: Snell RS, Lemp MA. *Clinical Anatomy of the Eye* (2nd Edition). John Wiley and Sons (1998).

28. B.

The abducens nerve has the longest intracranial course of all the cranial nerves. It emerges from the anterior surface of the brainstem, whereas the trochlear nerve is the only cranial nerve that emerges from the posterior surface of the brainstem. The abducens nerve passes through the superior orbital fissure within the common tendinous ring.

Further reading

Chapter 1: Anatomy of the eye and orbit. In: Forrester JV, Dick AD, McMenamin PG, Roberts F, Pearlman E. *The Eye: Basic Sciences in Practice* (4th Edition). Elsevier (2016).

Chapter 10: Cranial nerves—part 1: the nerves directly associated with the eye and orbit. In: Snell RS, Lemp MA. *Clinical Anatomy of the Eye* (2nd Edition). John Wiley and Sons (1998).

29. C.

The optic chiasm is approximately 12 mm wide and 8 mm long.

Further reading

Chapter 13: The visual pathway. In: Snell RS, Lemp MA. *Clinical Anatomy of the Eye* (2nd Edition). John Wiley and Sons (1998).

30. B.

The corneal and conjunctival epithelium, lens, and lacrimal and tarsal glands are all derived from surface ectoderm. The corneal stroma, sclera, iris, ciliary musculature, vitreous body, and choroid are all derived from mesoderm.

Further reading

Chapter 1: Development of the eye and the ocular appendages. In: Snell RS, Lemp MA. *Clinical Anatomy of the Eye* (2nd Edition). John Wiley and Sons (1998).

Physiology 5

Physiology of the eye and vision

31. D.

In healthy eyes, an average intraocular pressure of approximately 15 mmHg is generated by the flow of aqueous humour against resistance. The refractive index of aqueous humour is approximately 1.33. The concentration of ascorbate in aqueous humour is 20 times greater than that in plasma.

Further reading

Gabelt BT, Kaufman PL. Chapter 11: Production and flow of aqueous humor. In: Levin LA, Nilsson SFE, Ver Hoeve J, et al. *Adler's Physiology of the Eye* (11th Edition). Elsevier (2011).

32. D.

Reduced glutathione levels in whole lenses or lens epithelial cells can cause cell damage and cataract formation.

Further reading

Beebe DC. Chapter 5: The lens. In: Levin LA, Nilsson SFE, Ver Hoeve J, et al. *Adler's Physiology of the Eye* (11th Edition). Elsevier (2011).

33. B.

The secondary vitreous appears at the end of the sixth week of embryological development.

Further reading

Lund-Anderson H, Sander B. Chapter 6: The vitreous. In: Levin LA, Nilsson SFE, Ver Hoeve J, et al. *Adler's Physiology of the Eye* (11th Edition). Elsevier (2011).

34. A.

Docosahexaenoic is essential for renewal of the photoreceptor outer segments. It cannot be synthesised by the photoreceptors. It is synthesised in the liver from its precursor, linolenic acid. It is transported to the eye via the bloodstream, bound to plasma protein.

Further reading

Strauss O, Helbig H. Chapter 13: The function of the retinal pigment epithelium. In: Levin LA, Nilsson SFE, Ver Hoeve J, et al. *Adler's Physiology of the Eye* (11th Edition). Elsevier (2011).

35. B.

When the ciliary muscle contracts, the suspensory ligaments slacken and the lens capsule moulds the young lens into a more spherical form. During accommodation, the thickness of the lens cortex does not change, but the thickness of the lens nucleus increases. In 1909, Helmholtz described the accommodative mechanism of the eye, including increased anterior surface curvature and anterior movement of the anterior lens surface, but he did not describe posterior movement of the posterior lens surface, which has since been demonstrated.

Further reading

Glasser A. Chapter 3: Accommodation. In: Levin LA, Nilsson SFE, Ver Hoeve J, et al. *Adler's Physiology of the Eye* (11th Edition). Elsevier (2011).

36. C.

There are three types of cone photopigment: short-wavelength sensitive (S), middle-wavelength sensitive (M), and long-wavelength sensitive (L). These are maximally sensitive to wavelengths of 415 nm, 530 nm, and 560 nm, respectively.

Further reading

Neitz J, Mancuso K, Kuchenbecker JA, Neitz M. Chapter 34: Color vision. In: Levin LA, Nilsson SFE, Ver Hoeve J, et al. *Adler's Physiology of the Eye* (11th Edition). Elsevier (2011).

General physiology

37. D.

Sarcoplasm is the intracellular fluid that fills the spaces between myofibrils. It contains large quantities of potassium, magnesium, phosphate, multiple protein enzymes, and mitochondria. The mitochondria provide large quantities of adenosine triphosphate (ATP) to the myofibrils.

Further reading

Chapter 6: Contraction of skeletal muscle. In: Hall JE. *Guyton and Hall Textbook of Medical Physiology* (13th Edition). Elsevier (2016).

38. B.

When an action potential reaches the neuromuscular junction, voltage-gated calcium (not sodium) channels are activated. Acetylcholine vesicles fuse with the neural membrane and release acetylcholine into the synaptic cleft via exocytosis (not endocytosis). Neostigmine stimulates the neuromuscular junction by inhibiting (not activating) acetylcholinesterase.

Further reading

Chapter 7: Excitation of skeletal muscle: neuromuscular transmission and excitation. In: Hall JE. *Guyton and Hall Textbook of Medical Physiology* (13th Edition). Elsevier (2016).

39. C.

The pancreas contains 1–2 million islets of Langerhans. The acini secrete digestive juices directly into the duodenum. The alpha cells (25%) secrete glucagon, the beta cells (60%) secrete insulin and amylin, the delta cells (<10%) secrete somatostatin, the epsilon cells (<1%) secrete ghrelin, and the PP cells (<5%) secrete pancreatic polypeptide.

Further reading

Chapter 79: Insulin, glucagon, and diabetes mellitus. In: Hall JE. *Guyton and Hall Textbook of Medical Physiology* (13th Edition). Elsevier (2016).

40. C.

Vitamin B_1 (thiamine) deficiency causes gastrointestinal tract disturbances, weakens the heart, and causes peripheral vasodilation; severe vitamin B_1 deficiency causes cardiac failure. Vitamin B_{12} deficiency causes pernicious anaemia and demyelination of the large nerve fibres of the spinal cord.

Further reading

Chapter 72: Dietary balances; regulation of feeding; obesity and starvation; vitamins and minerals. In: Hall JE. *Guyton and Hall Textbook of Medical Physiology* (13th Edition). Elsevier (2016).

Biochemistry

41. D.

Mitochondria are approximately 2 micrometres long. They comprise a two-membrane compartment system. The mitochondrion inner membrane organising system (MINOS) is located at the cristae junction with the inner boundary membrane.

Further reading

Chapter 4: Biochemistry and cell biology. In: Forrester JV, Dick AD, McMenamin PG, Roberts F, Pearlman E. *The Eye: Basic Sciences in Practice* (5th Edition). Elsevier (2021).

42. D.

The corneal stroma accounts for approximately **90%** of total corneal thickness. Type I collagen accounts for approximately **55%** of stromal collagen. Stromal type I collagen is arranged in an **orthogonal** (i.e. at right angles) lamellar fashion.

Further reading

Chapter 4: Biochemistry and cell biology. In: Forrester JV, Dick AD, McMenamin PG, Roberts F, Pearlman E. *The Eye: Basic Sciences in Practice* (5th Edition). Elsevier (2021).

43. B.

UV-B light exposure is associated with an increase in cortical and posterior subcapsular formation, but not nuclear cataract formation. The ordered packing of lens crystallins is disturbed by increased water accumulation in the lens, vacuole formation within the lens fibres, and formation of high-molecular-weight lens protein aggregates.

Further reading

Chapter 4: Biochemistry and cell biology. In: Forrester JV, Dick AD, McMenamin PG, Roberts F, Pearlman E. *The Eye: Basic Sciences in Practice* (5th Edition). Elsevier (2021).

Pathology 5

General and ocular pathology

44. D.

Apoptosis is an active process involving cleavage of proteins by caspase enzymes.

Further reading

Chapter 9: Pathology. In: Forrester JV, Dick AD, McMenamin PG, Roberts F, Pearlman E. *The Eye: Basic Sciences in Practice* (4th Edition). Elsevier (2016).

45. D.

The growth of a neoplasm is progressive, has no regard for surrounding tissues, is unrelated to the body's requirements, and persists after the initiating stimulus has been withdrawn. Benign neoplasms are typically well circumscribed and slow growing. On the other hand, malignant neoplasms have ill-defined, irregular boundaries and can grow rapidly, demonstrating local and distant spread by invading body spaces, arteries, veins, and lymphatic channels. Malignant neoplasms can also undergo necrosis.

Further reading

Chapter 9: Pathology. In: Forrester JV, Dick AD, McMenamin PG, Roberts F, Pearlman E. *The Eye: Basic Sciences in Practice* (4th Edition). Elsevier (2016).

46. A.

In age-related macular degeneration (AMD), local ischaemia can occur due to increased production of extracellular matrix due to local inflammation. Inflammatory cells may then produce pro-angiogenic molecules including vascular endothelial growth factor (VEGF), which cause neovascular (wet) AMD.

Further reading

Chapter 9: Pathology. In: Forrester JV, Dick AD, McMenamin PG, Roberts F, Pearlman E. *The Eye: Basic Sciences in Practice* (4th Edition). Elsevier (2016).

47. A.

HLA-B51 is associated with Behçet's retinal vasculitis. HLA-DR4 is associated with Vogt-Koyanagi-Harada disease. HLA-B27 is associated with ankylosing spondylitis. HLA-A29 is associated with birdshot retinochoroidopathy.

Further reading

Chapter 9: Pathology. In: Forrester JV, Dick AD, McMenamin PG, Roberts F, Pearlman E. *The Eye: Basic Sciences in Practice* (4th Edition). Elsevier (2016).

48. B.

Anterior synechiae are adhesions that form between the peripheral iris and trabecular meshwork, while posterior synechiae form between the pupillary iris and lens. Pseudoexfoliation syndrome is the most common form of secondary open-angle glaucoma. Secondary closed-angle glaucoma is caused by the mechanical closure of the iridocorneal angle due to anterior displacement of the lens.

Further reading

Chapter 9: Pathology. In: Forrester JV, Dick AD, McMenamin PG, Roberts F, Pearlman E. *The Eye: Basic Sciences in Practice* (4th Edition). Elsevier (2016).

49. B.

Lattice corneal dystrophy is inherited in an autosomal dominant manner. Microscopy reveals amyloid deposit (see Table 1.6, p. xxx, and Fig. 1.8, p. xxx). It commonly recurs in grafts.

Further reading

Chapter 9: Pathology. In: Forrester JV, Dick AD, McMenamin PG, Roberts F, Pearlman E. *The Eye: Basic Sciences in Practice* (4th Edition). Elsevier (2016).

50. A.

Juvenile forms of optic pathway glioma carry a relatively good prognosis, while adult forms carry a relatively poor prognosis and are associated with extensive intracranial extension.

Further reading

Chapter 9: Pathology. In: Forrester JV, Dick AD, McMenamin PG, Roberts F, Pearlman E. *The Eye: Basic Sciences in Practice* (4th Edition). Elsevier (2016).

Helfferich J, Nijmeijer R, Brouwer OF, et al. Neurofibromatosis type 1 associated low grade gliomas: a comparison with sporadic low grade gliomas. *Critical Reviews in Oncology/Hematology.* 2016 Aug;*104*:30–41.

51. D.

Dermoid cysts can develop during embryogenesis, resulting from the incarceration of ectoderm between the frontal and maxillary processes; they contain pilosebaceous follicles and hair. Sudoriferous cysts (hidrocystomas) originate from the glands of Moll; they are lined by a double layer of epithelium. Epidermoid cysts can occur due to epithelial inclusion following surgery or trauma, or following obstruction of the duct of a pilosebaceous follicle; they are filled with keratin.

Further reading

Chapter 9: Pathology. In: Forrester JV, Dick AD, McMenamin PG, Roberts F, Pearlman E. *The Eye: Basic Sciences in Practice* (4th Edition). Elsevier (2016).

52. D.

Lacrimal gland tumours are locally aggressive and can invade surrounding structures if untreated.

Further reading

Chapter 9: Pathology. In: Forrester JV, Dick AD, McMenamin PG, Roberts F, Pearlman E. *The Eye: Basic Sciences in Practice* (4th Edition). Elsevier (2016).

Microbiology

53. D.

Bacillus cereus is a Gram-positive, rod-shaped, spore-forming bacterium. It is commonly found in soil and food. It does not represent normal ocular flora. It can cause endophthalmitis, typically associated with traumatic injury.

Further reading

Chapter 8: Microbial infections of the eye. In: Forrester JV, Dick AD, McMenamin PG, Roberts F, Pearlman E. *The Eye: Basic Sciences in Practice* (4th Edition). Elsevier (2016).

54. B.

Mucormycosis typically occurs in immunocompromised individuals or those with poorly controlled diabetes mellitus.

Further reading

Chapter 9: Pathology. In: Forrester JV, Dick AD, McMenamin PG, Roberts F, Pearlman E. *The Eye: Basic Sciences in Practice* (4th Edition). Elsevier (2016).

Immunology

55. D.

The innate immune system can be rapidly mobilised as it does not involve memory and is relatively non-specific. On the other hand, the acquired immune system has the following inherent characteristics: specificity, memory, specialisation, tolerance, diversity, and ability to downregulate.

Further reading

Chapter 7: Immunology. In: Forrester JV, Dick AD, McMenamin PG, Roberts F, Pearlman E. *The Eye: Basic Sciences in Practice* (4th Edition). Elsevier (2016).

56. A.

Cytokine pleiotropy describes the ability to exhibit multiple biological actions, whereas redundancy describes the exhibition of shared biological actions. Cytokines demonstrate both pleiotropy and redundancy They are short-lived and short-range molecules and can be effective at low concentrations. They can alter the effects of other cytokines and can induce cytokine synthesis themselves.

Further reading

Chapter 7: Immunology. In: Forrester JV, Dick AD, McMenamin PG, Roberts F, Pearlman E. *The Eye: Basic Sciences in Practice* (4th Edition). Elsevier (2016).

Pharmacology and genetics 5

Pharmacology

57. B.

Warfarin acts as a microsomal enzyme **inhibitor**. Other examples of microsomal enzyme inhibitors include metronidazole, chloramphenicol, and isoniazid.

Further reading

Chapter 6: General and ocular pharmacology. In: Forrester JV, Dick AD, McMenamin PG, Roberts F, Pearlman E. *The Eye: Basic Sciences in Practice* (5th Edition). Elsevier (2021).

58. B.

Pilocarpine is a parasympathomimetic. It facilitates aqueous outflow by direct action on the scleral spur and ciliary body.

Further reading

Chapter 6: General and ocular pharmacology. In: Forrester JV, Dick AD, McMenamin PG, Roberts F, Pearlman E. *The Eye: Basic Sciences in Practice* (5th Edition). Elsevier (2021).

59. D.

Topical steroids may cause a rise in intraocular pressure and secondary **open-angle** glaucoma, likely because of reduced aqueous outflow due to the accumulation of glycosaminoglycans and water in the trabecular meshwork.

Further reading

Chapter 6: General and ocular pharmacology. In: Forrester JV, Dick AD, McMenamin PG, Roberts F, Pearlman E. *The Eye: Basic Sciences in Practice* (5th Edition). Elsevier (2021).

60. A.

Azathioprine and mycophenolate (CellCept®) can cause bone marrow suppression and gastrointestinal upset. Ciclosporin and tacrolimus can cause nephrotoxicity, hypertension, hyperlipidaemia, glucose intolerance, gingival hyperplasia, and hirsutism. Corticosteroids can cause osteoporosis, hypertension, glucose intolerance, and altered habitus.

Further reading

Chapter 6: General and ocular pharmacology. In: Forrester JV, Dick AD, McMenamin PG, Roberts F, Pearlman E. *The Eye: Basic Sciences in Practice* (5th Edition). Elsevier (2021).

61. B.

Horner's syndrome is caused by an interruption of the sympathetic nervous supply to the eye. The classical triad of symptoms are **partial ptosis**, **anhidrosis**, and **miosis**. Partial ptosis is due to loss of sympathetic innervation of Müller's muscle. Anhidrosis (loss of sweating) with first-order lesions affects the ipsilateral side of the body, while with second-order neurons, anhidrosis affects the ipsilateral face, and with third-order neuron lesions, anhidrosis only affects a small amount of the face adjacent to the ipsilateral brow. Miosis is due to loss of sympathetic tone to the iris. Horner's syndrome can be associated with life-threating disease, such as dissecting aortic aneurysm or **superior** pulmonary sulcus tumour, also termed apical lung tumour or Pancoast's tumour.

Further reading

Chapter 6: General and ocular pharmacology. In: Forrester JV, Dick AD, McMenamin PG, Roberts F, Pearlman E. *The Eye: Basic Sciences in Practice* (5th Edition). Elsevier (2021).

62. D.

Apraclonidine and phenylephrine dilate postganglionic Horner's syndrome due to denervation hypersensitivity. Hydroxyamphetamine 1% causes the release of neurotransmitter from postganglionic fibres (third-order neurons), hence if affecting preganglionic fibres there is normal pupil dilation, whereas if affecting postganglionic fibres there is no dilation as no noradrenaline to release. Cocaine prevents the reuptake of noradrenaline, causing pupil dilation. There is no cocaine-induced pupil dilation in Horner's syndrome with the loss of sympathetic drive.

Further reading

Chapter 6: General and ocular pharmacology. In: Forrester JV, Dick AD, McMenamin PG, Roberts F, Pearlman E. *The Eye: Basic Sciences in Practice* (5th Edition). Elsevier (2021).

Genetics

63. B.

The four nucleotide bases in DNA are adenine (A), cytosine (C), guanine (G) and thymine (T). In mRNA, uracil (U) replaces thymine (T).

Further reading

Chapter 3: Genetics. In: Forrester JV, Dick AD, McMenamin PG, Roberts F, Pearlman E. *The Eye: Basic Sciences in Practice* (5th Edition). Elsevier (2021).

64. A.

The ribosome has two binding sites for transfer RNA (tRNA). The peptidyl-tRNA-binding site (P site) holds the tRNA and polypeptide chain. The aminoacyl-tRNA-binding site (A site) holds the incoming tRNA molecule. The stop codon on the messenger RNA causes binding of release factor to the **aminoacyl-tRNA-binding site (A site)**, which causes hydrolysation of the peptidyl-tRNA molecule on the P site and release of the polypeptide chain.

Further reading

Chapter 3: Genetics. In: Forrester JV, Dick AD, McMenamin PG, Roberts F, Pearlman E. *The Eye: Basic Sciences in Practice* (5th Edition). Elsevier (2021).

65. B.

Autosomal dominant inheritance is associated with **variable expressivity**. The same is true in X-linked recessive inheritance. Autosomal recessive inheritance is associated with constant expressivity.

Further reading

Chapter 3: Genetics. In: Forrester JV, Dick AD, McMenamin PG, Roberts F, Pearlman E. *The Eye: Basic Sciences in Practice* (5th Edition). Elsevier (2021).

66. D.

An epigenetic trait is a stably heritable phenotype caused by changes in a chromosome without alteration in the DNA sequence.

Further reading

Chapter 3: Genetics. In: Forrester JV, Dick AD, McMenamin PG, Roberts F, Pearlman E. *The Eye: Basic Sciences in Practice* (5th Edition). Elsevier (2021).

67. B.

COL2A1 mutation is associated with Stickler syndrome.

Further reading

Chapter 3: Genetics. In: Forrester JV, Dick AD, McMenamin PG, Roberts F, Pearlman E. *The Eye: Basic Sciences in Practice* (5th Edition). Elsevier (2021).

68. C.

Multifactorial inheritance can be categorised as continuous or discontinuous. Continuous traits demonstrate a **range** of disease expression, e.g. blood pressure. Discontinuous multifactorial traits demonstrate increased incidence in **affected families** compared to the general population. Some discontinuous multifactorial traits demonstrate **unequal** sex distribution, whereby the threshold for disease penetrance is lower in one sex than the other.

Further reading

Chapter 3: Genetics. In: Forrester JV, Dick AD, McMenamin PG, Roberts F, Pearlman E. *The Eye: Basic Sciences in Practice* (5th Edition). Elsevier (2021).

Investigations 5

69. C.

In the interpretation of Humphrey perimetry results, false positives typically indicate that the patient responds to the sound of the machine even when it does not present a light stimulus, and/or simply presses the response button too often (i.e. 'trigger-happy' patient). False negatives typically occur when the patient fails to respond to a brighter light stimulus presented at a location where they previously responded to a dimmer light stimulus (i.e. the patient is fatigued). Fixation losses typically occur when the patient looks away from the fixation target—these can be detected by periodically presenting the light stimulus in the physiological blind spot.

Further reading

Mollan SP, Calcagni A, Keane PA. Chapter 2: Investigations and their interpretation. In: Denniston AKO, Murray PI. *Oxford Handbook of Ophthalmology*. Oxford University Press (2018).

70. B.

The Roman numerals (0, I, II, III, IV, and V) represent the target size in mm^2, and each successive Roman numeral represents a fourfold increase in area. The Arabic numerals (1–4) represent the light intensity in apostilbs (asb), whereby each successive number is 3.15 times brighter (0.5 log unit steps). The lowercase letters represent additional minor filters where 'a' is the darkest and 'e' the brightest—each successive letter represents an increase of 0.1 log unit.

Further reading

Mollan SP, Calcagni A, Keane PA. Chapter 2: Investigations and their interpretation. In: Denniston AKO, Murray PI. *Oxford Handbook of Ophthalmology*. Oxford University Press (2018).

71. C.

Sodium fluorescein is **soluble** in water. Fluorescein is stimulated by blue light (approximately **490 nm**) and emits green light (approximately **530 nm**). Sodium fluorescein is 70–85% bound to plasma albumin.

Further reading

Mollan SP, Calcagni A, Keane PA. Chapter 2: Investigations and their interpretation. In: Denniston AKO, Murray PI. *Oxford Handbook of Ophthalmology*. Oxford University Press (2018).

72. D.

In FFA, a defect in the retinal pigment epithelium (RPE), such as RPE atrophy or macular hole, is most likely to cause a window defect. Leakage of dye at the macula can be caused by cystoid macular oedema (characteristic petalloid appearance) or other macular oedema. Leakage of dye at the disc can be caused by papilloedema, inflammation, and ischaemic optic neuropathy. Leakage of dye elsewhere can be caused by vasculitis, new retinal vessels, or choroidal neovascularisation.

Further reading

Mollan SP, Calcagni A, Keane PA. Chapter 2: Investigations and their interpretation. In: Denniston AKO, Murray PI. *Oxford Handbook of Ophthalmology*. Oxford University Press (2018).

73. A.

Spectral domain OCT can achieve axial resolution of 3–8 micrometres.

Further reading

Mollan SP, Calcagni A, Keane PA. Chapter 2: Investigations and their interpretation. In: Denniston AKO, Murray PI. *Oxford Handbook of Ophthalmology*. Oxford University Press (2018).

74. B.

Papilloedema is optic nerve head swelling associated with raised intracranial pressure. This patient has raised intracranial pressure associated with craniosynostosis (premature fusion of the cranial sutures). See Fig. 5.2 for comparison between the normal optic nerve head and papilloedema on OCT. Note the raised neuroretinal rim, obliteration of the optic cup, and anterior deflection of Bruch's membrane.

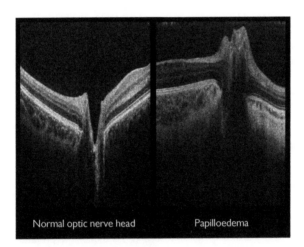

Normal optic nerve head   Papilloedema

Figure 5.2 Comparison between the normal optic nerve head and papilloedema on optical coherence tomography.

Adapted from: Rufai SR, et al. Feasibility and Repeatability of Handheld Optical Coherence Tomography in Children with Craniosynostosis. *Transl Vis Sci Technol*. 2021 Jul 1;10(8):24. CC BY 4.0.

Further reading

Mollan SP, Calcagni A, Keane PA. Chapter 2: Investigations and their interpretation. In: Denniston AKO, Murray PI. *Oxford Handbook of Ophthalmology*. Oxford University Press (2018).

75. D.

Standard fundus cameras typically deliver higher spatial and temporal resolution, as compared to SLO devices. Fig. 5.3 displays an ultra-widefield SLO image of the right retina, captured using the Optos® California (Optos plc, Dunfermline, UK).

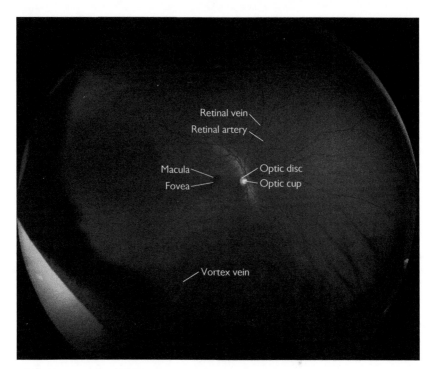

Retinal vein

Retinal artery

Macula

Fovea

Optic disc

Optic cup

Vortex vein

Figure 5.3 Ultra-widefield SLO image of the right retina.

Image courtesy of Mr Dermot F. Roche, Vision Scientist, Great Ormond Street Hospital for Children, London.

Further reading

Mollan SP, Calcagni A, Keane PA. Chapter 2: Investigations and their interpretation. In: Denniston AKO, Murray PI. *Oxford Handbook of Ophthalmology*. Oxford University Press (2018).

76. D.

Cerebrospinal fluid (a low-protein fluid) is bright on T2-weighted MRI but dark on T1-weighted MRI. By contrast, high-protein fluid is bright on T1-weighted MRI and dark on T2-weighted MRI. Air and dense bone are black on both. Fat is bright on T1-weighted MRI and moderately bright on T2-weighted MRI. Fig. 5.4 displays T1- and T2-weighted MRI head (coronal plane) for comparison. See also Fig. 4.3 (p. xxx) for basic orbital anatomy on a computed tomography angiogram.

Further reading

Mollan SP, Calcagni A, Keane PA. Chapter 2: Investigations and their interpretation. In: Denniston AKO, Murray PI. *Oxford Handbook of Ophthalmology*. Oxford University Press (2018).

77. B.

In full-field ERG, the a-wave primarily arises from photoreceptors hyperpolarising to light. The b-wave primarily arises from depolarising bipolar cells. Oscillatory potentials primarily arise from amacrine cells.

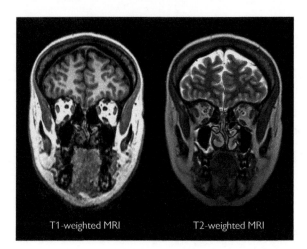

Figure 5.4 Comparison of T1-weighted (left) and T2-weighted (right) MRI.

Figure courtesy of Mr Aswin Chari, Clinical Research Fellow in Neurosurgery, Great Ormond Street Hospital for Children, London.

Further reading

Mollan SP, Calcagni A, Keane PA. Chapter 2: Investigations and their interpretation. In: Denniston AKO, Murray PI. *Oxford Handbook of Ophthalmology*. Oxford University Press (2018).

78. B.

Regarding the EOG, the normal LP:DT ratio is typically 1.7–4.3 with a light peak time ranging from 7 to 12 minutes.

Further reading

Constable PA, Bach M, Frishman LJ, et al. ISCEV Standard for clinical electro-oculography (2017 update). *Documenta Ophthalmologica. Advances in Ophthalmology*. 2017 Feb;*134*(1):1–9.

79. C.

The PERG provides an objective assessment of retinal macular function and distinguishes maculopathy from retinal ganglion cell/optic nerve disease. It utilises a reversing chequerboard to evoke PERG waveform features of prominent positive component at 50 milliseconds (P50) and a negative component at 95 milliseconds (N95)—note 'P' for 'positive' and 'N' for 'negative'. P50 is cone driven while N95 originates from the macular ganglion cells. The N95/P50 ratio is typically greater than 1.1. In addition to the N95/P50 ratio, amplitudes and peak times are evaluated when interpreting PERGs.

Further reading

Bach M, Brigell MG, Hawlina M, et al. ISCEV standard for clinical pattern electroretinography (PERG): 2012 update. *Documenta Ophthalmologica. Advances in Ophthalmology*. 2013 Feb;*126*(1):1–7.

Miscellaneous 5

80. B.

The SIGN classification can be used to grade levels of evidence. It can be summarised as follows:

1. Systematic review and meta-analysis, or randomised controlled trials.
2. Case–control or cohort studies.
3. Non-analytical studies (case reports/series).
4. Expert opinion.

The first two can be further subdivided according to quality and risk of bias—see SIGN classification for full details.

Further reading

Denniston AKO, Moseley M, Murray PI. Chapter 26: Evidence-based ophthalmology. In: Denniston AKO, Murray PI. *Oxford Handbook of Ophthalmology*. Oxford University Press (2018).

Scottish Intercollegiate Guidelines Network. SIGN 50: a guideline developer's handbook. 2019. Available at: http://www.sign.ac.uk/media/1050/sign50_2019.pdf Accessed October 2021.

81. D.

A Forest plot (or 'blobbogram') is used to display estimated results from several studies plus the overall meta-analysed measure of effect, which is represented by the dashed vertical line. The overall meta-analysed effect can also be plotted as a diamond whose lateral points indicate the confidence intervals. The solid vertical line represents the line of no effect. The size of the boxes indicates the individual study power (and therefore sample size) while the horizontal 'whiskers' indicate the confidence intervals per individual study.

Further reading

Denniston AKO, Moseley M, Murray PI. Chapter 26: Evidence-based ophthalmology. In: Denniston AKO, Murray PI. *Oxford Handbook of Ophthalmology*. Oxford University Press (2018).

82. D.

The median is the middle point of a data set, when arranged in ascending order. Fig. 4.4 (see p. xxx) summarises the data points displayed on a box and whisker plot. Please note that box and whisker plots can be orientated horizontally or vertically.

Further reading

Bunce C, Young-Zvandasara T. Simplified Ophthalmic Statistics (SOS). Part 2: how to summarise your data and why it's a good idea to do so. *Eye News*. 2018;*25*(2):34–35. Available at: https://www.eyenews.uk.com/education/trainees/post/sos-simplified-ophthalmic-statistics-part-2-how-to-summarise-your-data-and-why-it-s-a-good-idea-to-do-so Accessed October 2021.

83. A.

The World Health Organization recommends the ICD-11 definitions for distance and near visual impairment.

Distance visual impairment:

- Mild: visual acuity worse than 6/12 to 6/18.
- Moderate: visual acuity worse than 6/18 to 6/60.
- Severe: visual acuity worse than 6/60 to 3/60.
- Blindness: visual acuity worse than 3/60.

Near visual impairment:

- Near visual acuity worse than N6 or M.08 at 40 cm.

Further reading

World Health Organization. Blindness and vision impairment. 14 October 2021. Available at: https://www.who.int/news-room/fact-sheets/detail/blindness-and-visual-impairment Accessed October 2021.

84. A.

Fig. 1.10 (see p. xxx) is a flowchart displaying common statistical tests and rules.

Further reading

Bunce C, Young-Zvandasara T. Simplified Ophthalmic Statistics (SOS). Part 3: which statistical test should I use (if any)? *Eye News.* 2019;25(4):34–36. Available at: https://www.eyenews.uk.com/education/trainees/post/sos-simplified-ophthalmic-statistics-part-3-which-statistical-test-should-i-use-if-any Accessed November 2021.

85. B.

Fig. 1.10 (see p. xxx) is a flowchart displaying common statistical tests and rules.

Further reading

Bunce C, Young-Zvandasara T. Simplified Ophthalmic Statistics (SOS). Part 3: which statistical test should I use (if any)? *Eye News.* 2019;25(4):34–36. Available at: https://www.eyenews.uk.com/education/trainees/post/sos-simplified-ophthalmic-statistics-part-3-which-statistical-test-should-i-use-if-any Accessed November 2021.

86. D.

Fig. 1.10 (see p. xxx) is a flowchart displaying common statistical tests and rules.

Further reading

Bunce C, Young-Zvandasara T. Simplified Ophthalmic Statistics (SOS). Part 3: which statistical test should I use (if any)? *Eye News.* 2019;25(4):34–36. Available at: https://www.eyenews.uk.com/education/trainees/post/sos-simplified-ophthalmic-statistics-part-3-which-statistical-test-should-i-use-if-any Accessed November 2021.

87. C.

Selection bias can be caused by failure to achieve proper randomisation during participant selection. Recall bias can be caused by differences in the accuracy or completeness of recollections by participants regarding past events. Confirmation bias can be caused by the tendency to search for or favour information that confirms prior beliefs. Attrition bias can result from unequal loss of participants from different arms of a trial.

Further reading

Denniston AKO, Moseley M, Murray PI. Chapter 26: Evidence-based ophthalmology. In: Denniston AKO, Murray PI. *Oxford Handbook of Ophthalmology.* Oxford University Press (2018).

88. C.

Table 5.2 summarises the clinical trial phases and main goals.

Table 5.2 Clinical trial phases and main goals

Phase	Main goals
Preclinical	Drug testing in non-human subjects (*in vivo* and/or *in vitro*) to explore efficacy, toxicity, and pharmacokinetics with no dose restriction
0	Pharmacokinetics in ~10 humans using small, subtherapeutic doses
I	Dose-ranging in ~20–100 healthy human volunteers for safety
II	Drug testing at therapeutic dose in ~100–300 human patients with specific disease, to assess efficacy and side effects
III	Drug testing at therapeutic dose in ~300–3000 human patients with specific disease, to assess efficacy, effectiveness, and safety
IV	Post-marketing surveillance in public to monitor long-term effects (at therapeutic dose)

Further reading

US Food & Drug Administration. The Drug Development Process. 2018. Available online: https://www.fda.gov/patients/learn-about-drug-and-device-approvals/drug-development-process Accessed November 2021.

89. C.

Table 5.2 summarises the clinical trial phases and main goals.

Further reading

US Food & Drug Administration. The Drug Development Process. 2018. Available online: https://www.fda.gov/patients/learn-about-drug-and-device-approvals/drug-development-process Accessed November 2021.

90. D.

Table 5.2 summarises the clinical trial phases and main goals.

Further reading

US Food & Drug Administration. The Drug Development Process. 2018. Available online: https://www.fda.gov/patients/learn-about-drug-and-device-approvals/drug-development-process Accessed November 2021.

INDEX

For the benefit of digital users, indexed terms that span two pages (e.g., 52–53) may, on occasion, appear on only one of those pages.

Note: q indicates question; a indicates answer.

Tables and figures are indicated by *t* and *f* following the page number